Your Body Is Talking; Are You Listening?

Other Books by Art Martin

Mind/Body Medicine Connection:
Pscychoneuroimmunology in Practice
Becoming a Spiritual Being In a Physical Body
2011: The New Millennium Begins
Opening Communication with GOD Source
Recovering your Lost Self
Journey into the Light

Your Body Is Talking; Are You Listening?

The Mind/Body Medicine Connection:
Understanding the Theory of
Psychoneuroimmunology in the
Process of Healing
(with Case Histories)

Art Martin D.D. M.A.

Personal Transformation Press
A Division of the Wellness Institute

Your Body Is Talking; Are You Listening?
by Art Martin D.D. M.A.

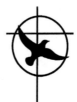

Published by
Personal Transformation Press
8300 Rock Springs Road
Penryn, CA 95663
Phone: (916) 663-9178
Fax: (916) 663-0134
Orders only: (800) 655-3846

This book explores the body/mind connection as the actual cause of all men-
tal/emotional dysfunction and physical disease. However, the author in no
way makes any diagnosis of medical condition or prescribes any medical treatment whatsoever.

Printed in the United States

Table Of Contents

Let There Be Peace On Earth

Let there be peace on earth
And let it begin with me.
Let there be peace on earth,
The peace that was meant to be.

With God as our one source
United all are we,
Let us walk with each other
In perfect harmony.

Let peace begin with me,
Let this be the moment now
With every step I take,
Let this be my solemn vow:

To take each moment
And live each moment
In peace eternally.

Let there be peace on earth
And let it begin with me.

— Anon

Dedication

This book is dedicated to all the
practitioners of Neuro/Cellular Repatterning
who learned the process and provided the support
to heal my body/mind, and all my sponsors who have
supported my work and helped me present
lectures, workshops and seminars

Acknowledgments

My first introduction to healing came in 1978 at an accupressure workshop taught by Iona Teagarden. That same year, I met Paul Solomon, who would be my teacher for the next ten years. He was my mentor and, along with Ronald Beesley, gave me a deep understanding of how healing works. I am indebted to them for starting me on the right path. In great physical pain at the beginning, I also worked with Frank Hughes, owner of Nance's Hot Springs in Calistoga, California, and am grateful for his intensive work with me.

I formed the Wellness Institute in Sacramento, California, and between 1984 and 1987, I began to incorporate hands-on therapy in my verbal counseling, and I thank those who let me experiment with the process I was developing: Body/Mind/Integration, later to become Neuro/Cellular Repatterning (N/CR). If it had not been for those who attended my classes and came to me as clients, none of this would have happened. I learned more from working with my clients than I ever did at a class or seminar.

When we closed the center, Chris Issel asked me if I would teach the process to a group. This landmark seminar proved to me that N/CR was not a special gift of healing I had; it was possible to train others to do the same thing. Suddenly, sponsors popped up everywhere as the original seven seminar attendees in turn set out to teach the technique. In a domino effect, Chris Issel introduced me to Jim Ingram, who turned out to be my major sponsor in Southern California, putting on workshops and introducing me to even more people. Many thanks to Jim and Chris for their invaluable support. Mary Best introduced me to Pattie Marshall, who offered to bring me to San Diego, and she took care of me as if I was her son. I thank her so much for getting me established in San Diego.

I am especially grateful to Amy Kinder, whose support went beyond what most people would offer. For many years, she set up clients and workshops and provided me a place to stay when I was in San Diego.

The list goes on; Helen Phelps, Joline Stone, Betts Richter,

Lesley Gregory, Joy Johnston, Oshara Miller, Nancy Worthington, Araya Lawrence, Ilene Botting, Robert Perala, Joyce Techel, Barbara Stone, Nadeen Gotlieb, Ruth Johnston, Sally Machutta, Karen Arnold, Mindy Cantor, Nicole Cooledge, Sherri Decker, Jim Dorobiala, Marilyn Grow, John Hammer, Marilyn Henderson, Bill Irwin, Barbara Ikeda, Jeane Joregensen, David Kamitzer, Kismit, Angel Kay, Susan Moulton, Morningstar Black, Kate Moyers, Janette Nash, Joan Noel, Oshana, Joy Polte, Terry Pierson, Jean Rossman, Rita Raimondo, Karla Spitzer, Sara Sherman, Krita Sheyk, Bertha Taylor, Dave Thompson, Susie Taylor, Janet Tully, Ro Thompson, David Weisman, Wally Wallace, Rebecca West, and Ken Peterson, one of the best examples of someone who took what I had when I first started and ran with it. He has supported my work in many ways and continues to inspire me to this day.

When the workshops got larger than I could handle alone, Mike Hammer came along. He seemed to be a natural for N/CR and quickly learned the process. I appreciate all the help he provided during his tenure with me.

With the help of my clients, Neuro/Cellular Repatterning continued to evolve over the years, thanks to all the people who allowed me to work with them. Everyone taught me the process by working with me. Without any formal training program for N/CR, I depended on the people who participated with me. For example, Bernard Eckes came to a 1993 workshop with the attitude that he could not learn the technique. He is now one of my research associates. I thank him for his perseverance in sticking with N/CR so that he could work with me in developing the process. With his help, we have now perfected N/CR to the point that we can clear and heal any dysfunction.

To spread our message to the public, I began presenting lectures and workshops at conferences and Whole Life Expos, and I appreciate the support my wife, Susie, gave me by spending countless hours running booths at the shows.

The help needed to get this book out came from Tony Stubbs, my editor and typesetter, who smoothed out my syntax and tied the book together. I really appreciate his support and help.

Preface

It is 1978, and I am surrounded by thirteen women in a healing workshop. (The nineties have seen a major upsurge in participation by men as more men allow their feelings and emotions surface.) I have just discovered the body/mind connection and realized that all dysfunction originates in the mind. This revelation will lead me to form my basic theory on illness and disease: that disease exists only if the mind allows it to infect the body, that disease is a *creation* of the mind, and that just as quickly as it allows disease and illness to be created, the mind can heal the result of disease.

I have just run headlong into a controversial area that is not accepted by doctors and medical research people, let alone the general public. However, I cannot prove my hypotheses since I have no documented evidence. Over the next two decades, I will amass documentation that proves that every illness, disease, physical and mental dysfunction is controlled by programs in the mind. I will discover that *there are no limitations, that anything can be corrected and healed, including genetic defects that one is born with, that every dysfunction is a lesson being presented to you.* Are you listening to the message?

The body/mind is a delicate, awesome machine that operates on a very rigid protocol, as does a computer. The computer jargon, "garbage in, garbage out," means that if erroneous data is fed in, the output will also be wrong. Similarly, every word our mind picks up is sensory input to its "database," and our mind interprets this input and places a value on the feeling or emotion before it files the information. How sure can we be that this input is accurate?

The results of addictions, mental dysfunction, pain, illness and disease can be traced back to earlier emotional trauma and how we were treated by our primary caregivers. Regardless of who this person was, you as a child had every right to be nurtured with love and affection. If you were not showered with unconditional love and acceptance, you felt rejected and abandoned. If this behavior continued, then you began to feel as though you were not acceptable.

Such programming may even have begun in the womb. My research has shown that three out of five children are rejected before they're even born. Of course, the parents may not consciously have rejected the child, or known that the fetus was picking up their thoughts, attitudes, interpretations, feelings and conversations. Few realize that a fetus can record and recognize communication about or directed at them. After the baby is born, it may not consciously understand all the communication it picks up, but its mind still interprets the data based on the programs already in its database. The auto-pilot is operating at high efficiency.

My personal journey revealed that my 17 years of 24-hour pain were caused by *in utero* and childhood programming. In 1978, when for the first time I was without pain, I was amazed to discover its source. But releasing the associated emotional trauma would prove to take 15 years. Having suffered cruelly for over 20 years, I know what pain is. I know that we set it all up. Prompted by my lengthy recovery, I developed a process that decreases healing time by a factor of 20. But why would people do this to themselves in the first place? This book answers that question.

Most of us do not listen to the messages we get from our body. So, as a result, it breaks down and we wonder why. Then, when we feel pain or are sick, we run to the "body mechanics," specialists trained to handle dysfunction, illness and today's diseases. Is this a good thing? I do not think so. Look at their track record. Has medical research found the causes and developed a cure for disease?

We spend incredible amounts each year on cancer research, yet have we found a cure? No, nor will we. AIDS, for example, is about total rejection of self. It is a non-selective immune system disorder, yet researchers think they can stop it with drugs. They poison people's bodies with chemotherapy, hoping the "cure" will kill the invading virus before it kills the patient. Is this the way to heal people?

AIDS patients need love and forgiveness, not drugs that suppress the symptoms. The medical profession does not teach love and forgiveness. It teaches fear—fear that there is no way out, but if you have the money or insurance, they will treat the symptoms for you. I have a totally different outlook, however.

Much about health, healing, disease and illness is simply not true. For example, most people accept that disease is hereditary, passed from generation to generation. This is patently false. Another myth is that there are contagious diseases. In fact, there are only contagious people, who will set themselves up to contract disease.

These myths stem from research by the medical establishment. Illness and disease do exist—that is not debatable. The question is, *why do they exist?* Will medical researchers come up with a cure in the future? I don't think so. They may come up with better ways to suppress the symptoms, but I don't think they will ever be able to eradicate disease, at least not with drugs and surgery.

My research has proved that each cell has its own blueprint that allows it to regenerate perfectly when the limitations that cause it to malfunction are removed. Each cell reproduces daily. Wounds and cuts heal without outside help. Yet why is it that some people have limited healing, while others heal much more quickly? I contend that it's all based on the limitations we place on ourselves.

Our mind controls our resistance to disease, and this sets the stage for a breakdown in our immune system. Viruses and disease-causing agents exist in us and all around us 24 hours a day, and when our resistance is low, we are susceptible to attack by virus and bacteria.

Diseases such as asthma or diabetes are caused by old programs. Clear the programs and the beliefs, and you clear the disease. Clearing does not just mask the symptoms but eliminates the program that drives the dysfunction.

Today, the medical establishment is worried that overuse of antibiotics is leading to resistant strains of bacteria and viruses. In fact, this has already happened with tuberculosis, and in England today, TB is a veritable 20th century plague. If we keep trying to sidestep the lesson, this trend will increase. You cannot fool your mind. Disease is caused by denial of a lesson. If we deny the lesson and try to sidestep it with an antibiotic to control or stop the symptom, the mind will find a way to render the drug ineffective and unable to control the symptom so that you *must* deal with the lesson.

People who have a healthy diet and outlook on life are less likely to contract illness. However, a good diet will not protect you from disease. It may help, but the mind controls the creation and the healing of disease. If we are able to release the programs that cause self-rejection and feelings of abandonment, along with the "I'm not alright" syndrome, we find that these people seldom accept sickness in their life. It is the acceptance of the dysfunction that causes the disease syndrome to begin. We could call it a "mind trip," since we have to accept that it is possible to contract disease before our body can create the symptom.

Through twenty years of research, I have developed a therapy process described as Neuro/Cellular Repatterning that reveals any dysfunction and triggers healing. This book describes what true healing is, and how spiritual psychology combined with the N/CR therapy process can help in clearing up physical and emotional dysfunction. Medical research terms the process "psychoneuroimmunolgy." (It's typical of the medical profession to tack a very complicated name to this process. I often wonder if they understand what it really is, but at least I'm thankful that they now recognize that the mind and body are connected.)

Therapy must use the integrated body/mind connection, plus a spiritual component to balance the total picture. Healing does not require a diagnosis, prescription drugs or surgery. Healing will happen when the mind and the body are aligned with the goal of wellness and responsibility is reclaimed. The cause of all dysfunction is lack of love and avoidance of responsibility for self. We have the answers in this book.

Art Martin
Penryn, California

Introduction

Neuro/Cellular Repatterning is a process that will heal any dysfunction, illness or disease; all that is required is that you overcome your doubt and skepticism about the power of the mind to heal the body at all levels. Even those who claim to accept holistic alternative healing practices can get caught up in the tenets of allopathic medicine and forget the programs that are installed in our mind.

This book avoids any description about spiritual growth, transmutation, transfiguration, soul recovery, evolution of the soul or ascension. You cannot begin spiritual work until you recover your lost self on a physical, mental and emotional level. You cannot put a roof on the house until you build a solid foundation and erect the walls. Many people want to leap over the emotional work and jump into spiritual work before they learn how to fly.

This book is about transformation of our life path, about building a solid foundation by clearing the denials that govern our lives. The denials will block the emotional pain and cause us to accept beliefs and interpretations which create illusions that we accept as our reality. The deeper we fall into denial, the more we live in fear and survival. When we accept pain as a reality we can do nothing about, we set ourselves up for rejection, abandonment and failure, yet do not even recognize it. As a result, we go through life believing we are on the path, yet we keep choosing people for friends, partners, employers and relationships who are duplicates of our parents because we have not cleared the lessons with our parents. Most people have yet to take the first steps on the path: letting go of judgment, manipulation, blame, control; the need for authority; not giving away personal power; and not being a victim. This must all be addressed before you can take the first step on the spiritual path.

I was looking for a healing process that would provide relief from the pain that I had experienced for the past 20 years. My goal was to heal myself; I had no inclination to develop a healing process that would create miracles on demand. If I had known that I would be presenting this process to the public and writing a book about it, I would have been scared beyond belief.

For me, the pain went on continually, sometimes intense, sometimes light, but never ending for 20 years, twenty-four hours a day. I attended many seminars and workshops on healing, only to discover that all of them were working only with symptoms. My pain would recede, only to come back just as intense. I finally realized that the practitioners were trying to actually heal people but all they were doing was releasing energy or emotional charge. Unfortunately this does nothing to prevent the program from activating the pain again and again.

In my work, I have participated in hundreds of miracle healings, but do not claim to be a spiritual healer, or any form of healer for that matter. In my initial arrogance, I even went so far as getting a vanity license plate: HEALER. But then I realized that there's no such a person as a healer and no longer have the plate. What I practice is not energy work, even though some people describe it as such. I am a "software" developer and "computer" programmer. I know the rules that cause healing to happen and I follow the process. By doing so, I facilitate healing for people who are committed to follow my direction.

I believe the presence of God is within us all. All you have to do turn it on, get all the programs lined up properly, and healing will happen. Healing is nothing more than rewriting and installing new programs in the mind's computers.

If someone is actually "healed," why does the dysfunction return? The answer is that the mind plays games with our perception. We want to release the pain so much that we may delude ourselves into believing that something was released, when, in fact, our mind created the illusion of release. The cause of the pain is still there, but since the charge driving the pain was released, it appears as if the situation has been cleared. The challenge is always to use *discernment* to recognize what the program is and not deny the actual cause.

Healing can take place if you can go through a total transformation process, releasing the base cause and the source program, and accepting a new reality. Doctors call this "spontaneous remission."

When I purchased my first computer in 1982, I began to understand how the mind processes information. The more I learned about computers, the more I began to compare the mind with computer technology and realized that we are a biomagnetic/electrical machine run by four networking computers linked to every cell in the body through the neurological system and the meridians. The body also communicates chemically through the blood vessels and capillary system by means of neuropeptides.

This may seem to be a crass way to describe a human being, but all we have to do is find the dysfunctional program and rewrite the software, and the body will heal itself.

As we shall see, the four computers networked together are:
1. The Conscious Mind
2. The Middle Self's Conscious Rational Mind and sub-personalities
3. Subconscious Mind and its database
4. Holographic Mind (soul level of the mind)

Until recently, I went along with all the groups that blamed "Ego" as the manipulator in a person's life. I have now discovered the awesome power of the Middle Self and the Conscious Rational Mind's auto-pilot and how it functions—it runs primarily on belief. One would assume that all the Conscious Mind does is input information into the mind, but we are discovering there is more to Conscious Mind. Conscious Rational Decision-Making Mind is the outer level of the Middle Self mind. Autopilot runs from a segment in this area of the mind.

The inner level of the Middle Self is driven by beliefs, programs and sub-personalities. It cannot see the future at all. It assumes that the future will be the same as the past, and is irrational in its desire to protect us. The only problem is that Inner Middle Self operates primarily from fear, it must be right and in control. Since it projects fear onto your Conscious Mind, you may accept the fear as real, and it becomes your reality. As a result, your operating system becomes based on an illusion. This operating system functions from the Conscious Rational Mind which you cannot control since it is autopilot.

All physical dysfunction is caused by the mind, the beliefs, and the programs it operates. If programs in the Subconscious Mind computer's database are unable to transmit the proper signals to the body, we have a breakdown in the system. If the operational programs that drive your life begin to malfunction, you can have any form of disease, illness or a behavior breakdown.

If your Conscious Rational Mind computer is not driving your life, you are running on auto-pilot, which means there is very little communication with the rest of the network, and your Conscious Rational Mind's auto-pilot and Middle Self's sub-personalities are running your life. They possess little discretion, and will accept any incoming theory or diagnosis without question. If you are not monitoring incoming sensory input, everything is written into data storage. Every thought, action or dialogue is sensory input to the database, and recorded exactly as it happens. All diseases and dysfunctional syndromes are controlled by beliefs and programs that are driven by a base cause which is recorded in the database. When you act on a belief or interpretation often enough, you create a program that will cause a situation to manifest in your life.

You may be operating from a program that was created without your consent or awareness. If so, how do you find the cause of the dysfunction? Removing the result, changing the vibration or just becoming aware of the cause is not enough. We have to release and clear the base cause and all of the patterns that are attached to it. In my case we tried them all, but couldn't permanently clear the program until we discovered that we had to rewrite it.

We recently found that the old programs were still surfacing, even though we thought we had rewritten them. We found that we had to locate the sub-personality, too. So we erased, the sub-personality that was being driven by the belief and the program. When we got down to the encrypted and encoded programs, we realized that the *mother factor* has a major effect on a person's life. Everything a mother thinks, feels or hears during her pregnancy is recorded in the *child's* cellular memory.

As we looked further into the programming, we found that most people were under the influence of "I'm not alright," self-rejection, and abandonment programs, and these can be so deeply imbedded that clearing takes many sessions. We found that the Middle Self created these programs based on interpretations it made on early childhood sensory input. These were created by feelings which may not have been accurate, but were recorded and became programs, anyway.

Based on my research and realizations, I began to understand why people function as they do in life—and it has nothing to do with what I learned about in Behavioral Psychology in college. It was quite an adventure into an uncharted field. I was venturing into an area where I was the only one to make claims that *all* illness and disease was created by the mind. Recent medical research has discovered that the mind controls our physical health.

As early as 1981, I started experiencing miracles but at the time, I could not make any longterm claims; I could not say, "This condition was cleared five or ten years ago and has not reoccurred." And, of course, many people simply didn't believe my statements, so I documented evidence and information on the many healing "miracles" that have happened over the last 20 years.

I have also maintained contact with many of my early clients. Almost all have had a complete release of dysfunctional pattern or disease, what doctors would call "spontaneous remission." The only difference between healing and curing (or spontaneous remission) is that we never really know if the disease, illness or dysfunctional behavior will return. Many times, it reemerges in another form.

By rewriting the programs and releasing the base cause, we achieve total healing. Many people have turned their lives around and pulled out of a downward spiral. There appears to be no limitation on what can be cleared and healed once the program driving the belief or interpretation is removed. Ten years ago, programs occasionally recurred because we didn't understand the power of the Middle Self and blamed it on Ego, but with new understanding of how sub-personalities function, we can now achieve total clearing of a pattern. Since the advent of the recovery movement with John Bradshaw *et al*, it has been much easier for me to describe childhood problems and the continuing effect on adults until the trauma is released.

Since starting out, I have adjusted my original viewpoint on what healing is. Many people would contend that healing happens to some and not others, with no reason why. I assumed that was true because that's what happened to me. Some people would even state that "God was working with that person." That seemed to me like favoritism. The presence of God is in all of us. Unfortunately most people have their "God-switch" turned off due to overshadows that block them off from God. I know for sure that there is no favoritism in God's realm. Nobody is condemned, everybody has access to God's love. Miracles do happen; we are the only ones who block them. As Pogo (in the cartoon) said, "We have found the enemy and he is us."

I also had to readjust my view of psychological counseling. When I was a "talk therapist," many clients came back to me disappointed, feeling that situations we had cleared had retrenched themselves. It was frustrating for both of us to clearly outline the path they should take and then watch them sabotage themselves.

At this juncture, I questioned whether this was the path I wanted to take. Talking with one of my colleagues, I became even more frustrated when she said that on questioning her mentor psychologist, he described his practice in this manner: "About 30 percent of the people get it and change. 35 percent of the people may feel better, but it's hard to see any major long term changes in their life. And 35 percent don't get it at all, quit therapy, and go on living the role of victim as if they have no options."

With my own feelings of self-rejection coming up all the time, it was hard to see my way clear. I needed the validation of helping people, but if the failure rate was that high, was this the right path?

Rather than give up, I decided to change my practice because I was getting some amazing results with a new therapy process that a number of clients consented to try. When I ran into a challenge, I asked if the client would like to explore a new approach: the body/mind connection. If they were willing to try, we cleared it.

Some people were not comfortable with hands-on therapy. Many people want the therapist to simply commiserate with their problems. I am not interested in the soap operas that people call their lives. My work is to help people empower themselves, to help them recognize they have given their power away to people, situations, and programs. I want to help them reclaim their personal power, and take control and responsibility for their life.

As a result, I shifted my whole practice over to a combination of integrated body orientation and spiritual psychology. With this new body/mind process, I showed the client where the program was embedded in the body. In doing so, I discovered that healers do not exist. We heal ourselves. Indeed, *you* are the only one who *can* heal you. I realized we can only show clients the way. They must heal themselves. We can only be facilitators.

I also found that some people do not want to heal themselves since they're getting too much mileage out of being sick or dysfunctional. They get too much support for the "soap opera" drama in their lives. If you want people to take care of you and serve you, there are many benefits from being nonfunctional. Manipulating people into satisfying your needs also gives you a feeling of control and outer validation.

When you want to get on with your life, being unable to get to the root of some dysfunction can be frustrating. Failures in healing can take a high toll on you if you are getting your validation from outside yourself. I find this as one of main stumbling blocks in healing. We are defeating and sabotaging ourselves by looking for acceptance by others and striving for their conditional love. Having to take responsibility and not blaming someone else prevents you from reclaiming your personal power.

Knowing what the situation is and discussing it will not change the basic reality of behavior; my challenge is to get a client to understand that statement. We can set up a basic format which will cause healing, but will it be permanent? Many times, the situation or dysfunction will come back and recreate the same results if the program is not cleared and released. Many times we have to write new "software" to replace the program that was released.

A few researchers understand the scientific response to healing energy but very few have been able to duplicate it in a double blind test. Displacing, suppressing, controlling or removing the symptoms does not cure anything, but merely displaces the symptom and causes temporary remission.

I am committed to total healing so that the illness, disease, or mental or emotional dysfunction is eliminated and erased totally. This can and does happen all the time; this book offers many such case histories.

Healing is transmitted to the cellular level of the body by neuropeptides and cytokinins, and this causes a shift in the electrical transmission cycle. During the healing process, the energy transfer can increase to 50,000 to 100,000 Hz (cycles per second). The energy of healing shows clearly on an oscilloscope as a standing wave. This intense electrical potential causes a DNA shift that can only be described as a miracle. But if we're dealing with a machine that operates like a computer, why doesn't it happen every time? We have to go back to the programming to see if there is a limiting pattern built into the computer "software." If there is, then the computer is operating perfectly according to its programs.

One often hears a talk show host tell a caller to simply stop being driven by an addiction, obsession, or compulsive behavior. However, those who have not experienced overwhelming compulsion cannot and must not judge another person's behavior. People in denial of the illusion they are living will not be able to even discuss it with you. Most people who recognize the behavior pattern want to stop it, yet seem unable to do so. We cannot stop a compulsive pattern without getting to the base cause that is driving the belief or the program. Many people in recovery will trade one addiction for another compulsive or obsessive behavior. The mind must have an outlet for feelings that have to be satisfied, even if it is driven by an illusion.

Disease is a final result of emotional trauma. All cellular structures in the body are in constant contact with each other, the brain serving as the telephone operator. The power of the mind is unlimited. It can regenerate any dysfunction that begins in the mind, but it can also perfectly reconstruct any part of the body from each cell's blueprint of how it was created.

The body's bio-electromagnetic field must be totally balanced before we can begin to function properly. The body/mind operates with electric impulses. Blocked electrical transmission causes breakdowns in the body. When I discovered that we could readjust the body function by reprogramming the mind, I suddenly saw how healing happens.

The main conflict lies in the illusions and denial that are put up as smokescreens to block awareness of emotional trauma. Change by the mind will be blocked until awareness of the dysfunction is accepted. The challenge is to get all the sub-personalities in the inner, irrational Middle Self to go along with the Conscious and Subconscious Minds, and agree on a plan. When all your selves become aligned, healing can begin to take place, but until then, the mind seems to be split, with one side working against the other, causing a double-bind.

Our mind will intentionally cause a breakdown and disease in the body to protect us from the illusionary fear that it senses from the past. Middle Self, or a sub-personality, holds a belief that prevents us from doing something that it believes would cause us harm. It does not see that it is causing a problem that may be worse than the situation it is trying to avoid.

When we release the double bind, healing can begin to take place. Miracles do happen. All we have to do is get to the base cause, release it, and rewrite the script. In early 1997, we located the cause of many situations that we were unable to break through: you have multitudes of sub-personalities who will control your life with driving beliefs, attitudes and interpretations that are tied to habit patterns. When you clear and delete their operating system, they are no longer functional. The habit pattern, belief or program they are controlling will disappear, eliminating the reaction.

I know that each time I am confronted with a challenge, I will be given a method to deal with the situation and we will clear the trauma. There seems to be no limitation on what can be cleared and healed.

Chapter 1

The Body/Mind As a Vehicle for Personal Transformation

Everybody would like to live in happiness, joy, harmony and unconditional love; that was my goal, too. So why do we continue to follow a path that doesn't provide peace, happiness, harmony and joy?

Most of the time, we feel that if we have a concept down and a goal clearly in our mind, we can accomplish the task. In my research, I have found that most people put honest effort into changing their attitudes and behavior so as to reclaim their self-esteem and self-worth. But many do not seem able to accomplish their goal, so they become discouraged, frustrated and disappointed.

When we evaluate what's needed to empower ourselves, to change our path, to reclaim our self-esteem, we overlook the fact that our belief systems, along with our Conscious Irrational Middle Self coupled with Subconscious Mind, are very powerful. The challenge is that we may have the concept down in our Conscious Rational Mind, but we must have acceptance from *all four* minds (see Chapter 6 for a detailed description of the minds.)

I have found that Conscious Mind must be aligned with the Subconscious and the Instinctual Minds, or you will be sabotaged. However, you will be unable to "see" the situation until you can recognize it and believe it.

If you suppress or stuff your feelings, an illusion or denial will block your recognition of a problem situation. If you deny the problem, it does not exist in your reality. Of course, that doesn't mean that the situation *doesn't* exist; it just doesn't exist for *you*. It still exists separate from your willingness to recognize it.

Young children have little or no control over how their primary caregivers' treatment impacts them, and they form their beliefs in reaction to that early treatment. The programs thus laid down continue throughout our life, or until we change them. We lose our self-esteem and "alrightness" by giving away our personal power and allowing others to control how we feel. Few parents realize they are teaching negative emotions of rejection, disapproval, scolding, shame, guilt, and fear.

Some children are so sensitive to how they are treated or what is said that their lives can be programmed for failure or success. As a result, they may relinquish their personal power and begin to reject themselves, *even before their first birthday*. By their third year, many children have already set up their life path to become self-destructive or self-supportive. If this happens often, we separate ourselves from Source. When we experience separation from the presence of God within, we separate ourselves from our pipeline to unconditional love.

Many people have an illusion that any focused and concentrated form of attention is love, even physical abuse, and for healing to occur, their idea of love must be reestablished. I have found that over 85 percent of my clients do not love themselves. Becoming "all right" with themselves requires unraveling the negatives created by isolation, rejection, frustration, discouragement, disappointment, fear, invalidation, guilt and humiliation. We can attempt to give others praise, strokes, support, recognition for empowerment, and try to help them to recover their self-esteem and self-worth, but many will discount and reject such validation if they feel they're not worthy of it.

Contrary to popular belief, self-esteem is not learned. It is not something you can teach someone. We all have positive self-supporting qualities at birth, as well as the ability to experience happiness, joy and harmony. We are born in love and joy, not in sin as many religious people would have us believe. As we grow up, our perceptions and interpretations of how we were treated by our primary caregivers begin to shape our beliefs and our view of reality. We do not lose our self-esteem, self-worth and self-confidence; they are overwritten by our experiences as a child. Our perception of self either destroys or enhances our "self" qualities.

To compile a "Self-worth Inventory," we must look at the qualities that make us feel all right with ourselves. I use the term "alrightness" to encompass all the positive cluster qualities that give us the ability to feel and claim our self-esteem. For the purposes of listing them, I have separated them, but generally, if we have one, we will usually have them all:

1. *Self-Esteem:* feeling good about yourself with no need for external validation or approval.
2. *Self-love:* ability to recognize, support, respect, trust ourselves, and take responsibility, knowing you are all right without outside support. You empower yourself to be kind and caring of self, following a wellness program such as exercise and eating properly, listening to and respecting your body.
3. *Self-Confidence:* You know that you have the ability to accomplish your goals; you take responsibility for them.
4. *Self-approval:* You do not need anyone's approval or sanction to know that your actions are acceptable.
5. *Self-acceptance:* You can be happy without another person's love, support or acceptance.
6. *Self-validation:* You are all right. Nobody has to validate you or tell you that you are all right or loved.

Seldom do we know the base causes of any dysfunction in our lives. The body is a vehicle that will always tell you your history and the truth. Every sensory input has been stored in your cellular memory. Your subconscious mind's video/audio recorder has recorded every incident, reaction and response that ever happened to you, along with actual voice and pictures in absolute accuracy; nothing is ever overlooked, discarded or deleted.

Figure 1 shows that we can deal with conflict in our lives in one of two ways:
- Defensive and closed, which leads to the intent to protect against anticipated pain and fear, or
- Non-defensively and open, with the intent to learn from the conflict:

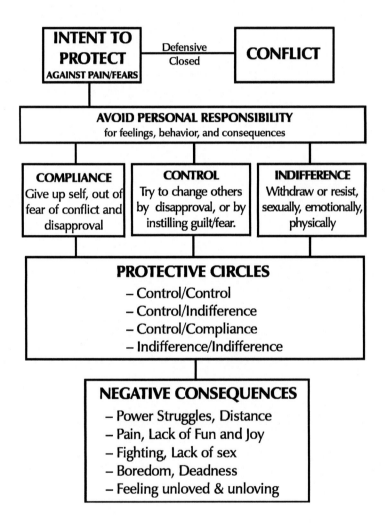

Figure 1: Dealing with conflict in our lives

With low self-esteem, and self-worth eroded by a negative environment, our primary motivation is the avoidance of future pain. We employ three main strategies:

- We comply out of fear of retribution and disapproval, which can lead to a "see-saw" of control behavior and retraction

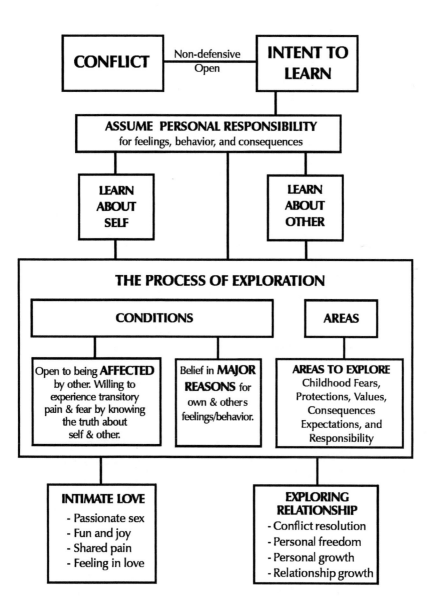

- We try to manipulate others by instilling guilt in them, as in "You'll be sorry when I'm dead or when I run away from home."
- We withdraw, which can lead to sullen, unresponsive behavior.

In all strategies, we develop mechanisms to cope with outer rejection of us, and the negative consequences of our coping mechanisms, such as fighting with siblings, meaningless activities such as "hanging out," and appearing as though nothing matters.

On the other hand, with self-esteem and self-worth intact, we are eager to learn about the world and how we can best interact with it. We take responsibility for our actions and their consequences, seeing life as a learning experience. This leads to three main areas of exploration:

- Ourselves and other people, accepting any transitory pain that may result as part of the rich tapestry life.
- Why we and others act and feel as we do, and seeking the reasons behind what happens.
- Areas such as childhood, fears, expectations, and personal responsibility.

This openness leads to being able to share love in intimate relationships, accepting them as arenas in which to resolve conflicts and explore personal freedom, the overarching goals being growth of self, other, and the relationship.

Chapter 2

Listening to the Messages Your Body/Mind Will Reveal

This book is based on a commitment to let the Body/Mind tell us the story of people's life history and how we can rewrite the scripts on which they live those lives. Some may find the following concepts and theory controversial, even unacceptable, but they come from twenty years working with clients as documented in case histories, rather than from book-based psychology. Some of these cases are described further in Chapter 14, but since some clients opted not to have their particular cases revealed, these are limited to those people who allowed me to write about their case.

The basic path of our life is planned before we even enter the body. Life can be compared to a crossword puzzle. All the open squares are free choice and the black squares are lessons we have to learn. As we fill in the puzzle of our life, we may decide to avoid the black squares and duck the lesson. We may even get into the lesson and call for a time out. The catch here is that we have only have a limited number of time outs in our life, and when we've used them all up, we have to "go for the goal" as they say in football.

Avoiding the minor lessons will usually cause discomfort, unhappiness, lack of love and abundance in our lives. But, if we choose a detour or denial to block a major lesson, we may instead manifest a severe, even life-threatening, disease or illness.

However, if we seek out the lessons and reclaim our personal power, we may experience discomfort at times, but we will achieve peace, happiness, harmony, joy and unconditional love and acceptance in our life.

How Do We Choose Our Path In Life?

Your life path is a macrocosm, covering many thousands of years, during which you make great strides and many mistakes, which, in turn, create Karma that you can balance in future lives. You choose the place and the time to work out the lessons, and you have as long as you need to do a thorough job. The progress you have already made in the past allows you to make more effective choices in future lifetimes. Belief, or otherwise, in reincarnation is irrelevant, since the cycle of return is a universal law. You know this at the soul level, and will continue to return until you finish the journey. For more information on these subjects, see my books *Being A Spiritual Being In a Physical Body* and *Journey Into the Light*.

Choosing Your Family Of Origin

Before birth, you as spirit choose your parents for the lessons you want to learn from them; they do not choose you. However, parents *can* influence the child to be born by reading material and meditating on the qualities that will attract an evolved soul. For example, in one Idaho family, the father was a potato farmer with barely a high school education, and the mother was a Korean war bride from a very poor background, also with little education. They had three children, two of whom were genius level students, and all of whom attended college on scholarships (the parents did not have the income to send even one of them to college).

The oldest child graduated from high school at 14 and left graduate school at 19 with a Ph.D. The second finished school almost as quickly. The third graduated in the normal timeframe, with honors and also went on to earn a Ph.D. All three found very good positions in industry.

Their mother had programmed these children by teaching herself English, and then reading from the Bible and many scholarly magazines and books. She admitted that she didn't understand much of what she read when she began her program. My wife and I undertook similar measures, and we turned out two intelligent, well-adjusted sons.

Unfortunately, most parents just start a family with no thought as to who they are attracting as a child. At the time of your conception, your body had a defect-free set of programs and blueprints to produce a perfect body. The lessons you wanted to learn and the lessons your parents had to learn from you determined the final result in the body you were born with. It may seem that you had no control over the defects that may be in your body at birth, but you were in total control of the outcome based on the choices you made prior to birth.

Many of my clients with genetic defects have been able to totally release, heal and correct them, so I know that the clients created the lessons during the pregnancy from the "flight plan" that they filed when they chose to enter this life.

Consider the case of a couple who delay having children until they graduate from college. The husband receives a good position as an instructor in the Department of Journalism of a well known university. After a few years, they have accumulated significant wealth and decide to have a child.

They are meditation and dream interpretation instructors, and as soon as the wife is pregnant, the husband begins a dialogue with the soul that has chosen to come to them. This soul already knows much about how their lives will unfold, and describes what will happen once he is born, and the nature of the lessons they will have to learn, but without revealing what the lessons are.

The soul tells them he will be a boy and what his name will be. They do not like his choice of name but go along with it since he is so accurate in his description of their lifestyle. The events that he describes for their future are upsetting, so they check in meditation with their Source to see if this is true. It is all validated, which upsets them more. They now know what will happen, but not how to stop it or deflect it.

The soul tells them he will become seriously ill when he is six months old. If they do not get the lesson, he will drop back below his birth weight and die. He adds that when he is 18 months old, he will have another medical emergency and the father will lose his job. If he does not get the lesson, they may both die. The father begins to doubt all this because he is healthy, follows a good dietary program, and exercises daily. He begins to lose confidence but, in other areas, the information is getting more definitive, so he continues the dialogue.

The dialogues stop when the child is born, but what the soul predicted happens right on schedule. At six months, the infant begins to lose weight and drops below his birth weight. As the soul had predicted, doctors cannot find anything medically wrong him. Their physician refers them to a homeopathic doctor who has come up with miracle cures in the past, yet officially, the physician disapproves of him. The homeopath is unable to help, but refers them to Paul Solomon, a medium who does readings in the style of Edgar Cayce. Solomon tells them to feed the child raw goat's milk, mixed half-and-half with lime water. This makes no sense at all to the parents, but it's all part of the lesson they have to learn, so they follow the direction and the child begins to gain weight.

After two months, the state in which they live passes legislation stopping the sale of any kind of raw milk, so they switch to pasteurized goat's milk and their son begins to lose weight again. They unsuccessfully scour health food stores for raw goat's milk. The homeopathic doctor knows of a farm that sells raw goat's milk, but warns, "You are perfectionist clean freaks, and although the dairy is sanitary, do not be shocked at what you see. This may be your lesson."

On entering the farm, they are appalled. As they approach the front door of the house, a goat walks out. Cats and dogs run loose all over the place. As they get out of their car, two goats come up to them like dogs looking for attention. They consider leaving, but know it's the only source of raw goat's milk in the area.

A lady comes out of the house, and in conversation, she tells them about her situation. She married right out of high school and they had several children, but then her husband had her declared incompetent as a mother, put her on disability, won custody of her children, and ran off with them. She has not seen them since. Without skills or training, when the disability payments ran out, she had no way to earn a living. She wanted to stay in the countryside since she hated the city, so she made her mind up and focused on what she wanted. She also let go of withholds and limitations on being willing to receive what comes along. As a result, a friend gave her some goats and the farm to manage. She considers the goats her children and treats them as such. The goats she raises for sale and for milk provide her a good income now that raw milk is banned, and the county inspectors overlook what she's doing since it keeps her off welfare. She and the parents become a good friends and they began helping her in her journey.

For the next five years, the story unfolds exactly as the soul predicted. They have many hard lessons to overcome because they come from a rule-controlled, compulsive family that has to have everything clean and perfect. But they learn to be more laid back and take life in stride. When the son is old enough to talk, they are amazed that he is able remember everything since birth.

Children up to six years old, who adults would not consider very aware, say the oddest things. One client told me that her four-year-old daughter said, "Mom, when I was your mother, I took better care of you than you're doing for me." The story checked out under regression.

In another case, a young girl called her grandmother "Mom," and her mother "Diane." It turned out that the grandmother was supposed to have been the little girl's mother but had an abortion at 34. This child was committed to clear this lesson with her would-be mother, now grandmother.

Some children are aware and can control the situation to some extent. Two children raised in the same manner will respond differently depending on the lessons agreed between them and their parents.

You get to choose how you respond or react to how your parents treated and raised you. You can be a survivor or a victim. No matter how mistreated and abused, survivors will eventually take control of their lives and succeed. On the other hand, victims may suffer much less or not at all, yet will claim some minor abusive treatment that they blame for their failure in life. Victims always have excuses to justify their failure.

You made the choice prior to entering this life, but you have probably lost the directions and the check list you made for your flight. You may remember why you're here, or may not know until you pass on out of this life. Unfortunately, after-death hindsight does not count toward evolution.

Granted, if you were raised in a functional family, you will have fewer problems in succeeding in life. But how did you choose this family of origin? It all has to do with the intentions you built into your prenatal flight plan and progress made during the lessons you presented to yourself in past lives. You start each life exactly where you left off when you left the previous one. The level to which you aspire in this life determines the type of parents you choose and their genetic background, so your choices also govern your body makeup and your physical attributes.

A sad fact I've discovered from the thousands of clients I've worked with in the last 20 years is that three out of five children were rejected before they were born, and one in five was rejected after birth. Thus only one person in five gets a fair start in life. Further, only one person in fifty comes from a family functioning well enough to make a real success out of life.

Almost half my female clients did not want children, yet most had them anyway, mainly due to erroneous programming installed by the church and parents, plus the basic societal/religious dogma that has overlaid our society for centuries. So, by far the greatest cause of our problems today is rejection and abandonment.

When a soul realizes that its choice of family was a mistake, it has two choices.

- If it decides not to proceed, it can chose not to enter the body, resulting in stillbirth.
- If it perceives that this will be rough on the family, it may accept that it made the choice to learn the lessons and opt to continue. Later on, if the child's life becomes too unbearable, the soul may "walk out," resulting in a crib death or some form of respiratory failure Very seldom do medical doctors find a reason, even though they will assign a cause of death. In my case, I had two near death experiences trying to back out of my family.

Choosing Your Race

Whether we like it or not, there is a pecking order in today's world, in which some races are subjected to more poverty and suffering than others. Of course, no one race is superior to another, and it has been proven over and over that people can succeed no matter what their origin. We choose our race based on what we want to learn, and every soul must undertake lives of subjugation and oppression, just as much as lives of mastery and dominion.

Western cultures have been trying to level the racial playing field for the last fifty years, but it will not work in the long run since we must have choices in learning certain lessons.

Choosing Your Gender

Gender is probably the most controversial issue all. To preface this section, over 20 years ago, when first getting into the human potential and spiritual awareness movement, I worked with

Tara Singh, a teacher, who said something that boggled my mind at the time: "You will never teach anything you have not had direct experience with. If you try to teach something that is not your direct experience, *it will become your experience* by virtue of having to learn it through some situation forcing its way into your life." That is exactly what has happened to me in many situations, including the sensitive issue of choice of gender.

Gender is obvious with heterosexuals. You are clearly male or female, with no question as to your identity. Of course, some men feel that women have an easier ride, which can cause envy and resentment. And many women feel they have to compete in a "man's world."

A number of my clients with breast cancer blame their bodies, saying that if it weren't for their breasts, the cancer would not have occurred. Some go so far as to curse their bodies and reject their femininity.

Many men fear women emasculating them or taking their power away, and may develop prostate or testicular cancer. The overwhelming need for sexual identity in the U.S. today is causing much dysfunction in the population, compounded by denial, a topic explored in depth in a later chapter.

Later chapters explore how our minds work, and how, unknown to us, our lives are controlled by programs stored in our minds until we reclaim our personal power and regain control over the direction of our life. With both the men and women above, the problem is rejection of the self.

Probably the most controversial question is, "Are people born with a sexual proclivity?" At one level, the answer is yes, in that we are born with male or female "plumbing." The only glitches are that we can carry programs over from past lives, and that the way our parents raise us can conflict with our plumbing.

You can bring a genetic disposition from past lives that will tilt you toward the gender with which you are most familiar. The mind, being a computer, records everything from your first incarnation onwards.

How your gender was treated in past lives will also create a predisposition. However, in 20 years of practice, I encountered only two men who were homosexuals based on past Karma in that they chose to experience homosexuality to deal with lessons they created in past lifetimes. Once we cleared the lessons, they chose to live as heterosexuals.

Historically, same-gender attraction moves in and out of favor. In ancient Roman and Greek cultures, homosexuality was the preferred basis for meaningful relationships, with heterosexuality relegated to mere procreation. And in today's Western world, it enjoys increasing acceptance by many people.

I have worked with many people in same-gender relationships and this chapter reports my findings. Sexual orientation is a matter of free choice, and I have no opinion either way, nor do I side with one position or another. My only concern is helping clients overcome the obstacles that block them from peace, harmony, happiness, joy, unconditional love and acceptance in their lives. Any judgement or opinion in the following is purely that of clients who perceive that their orientation is the source of such a block in their lives.

Every client I've worked with has an "original cause" program that directs them to make the life decisions that in turn cause them to make the lifestyle choices they do. This original cause is directly tied to a "base cause" which in turn will be triggered by catalyst situations that initiate the program and whatever habit pattern was laid down in the past (more about this in later chapters).

Now suppose your soul determines that you need a certain kind of person in your life to provide an experience it needs to learn from. Your soul will ensure that you are attracted to a person of that type. In fact, you both made a pre-life agreement to participate in the learning experience. The other person's gender may or may not be relevant. You can have just as abusive a relationship (as either abuser or abusee) in a same-gender relationship as you can in a male/female one.

Many clients have had a series of abusive male/female relationships, beginning with their mother or father, and continuing through young adult to one or more failed marriages. So they turn to same-sex relationships in hopes that the verbal abuse will stop, yet it doesn't. When we clear the original cause and the lesson attached to it, the catalyst and the program can no longer be triggered. So when the client meets new people who do not have the matching behavior pattern, the abuse pattern no longer occurs.

What drives people into same-sex relationships? Many of my lesbian clients are driven by anger or fear. Most dominant lesbians are driven by anger at men, which can usually be traced back to a strong, controlling father. A woman who may have been sexually molested by an abusive father or male relative may grow up to hate the father image, or angry at all men.

Parents' expectations (even subconscious) that a daughter should have been a boy can place a definite male energy overlay on the young girl, which can cause gender misidentification. How the daughter is treated and brought up can reinforce or erode the condition.

Passive women in a lesbian relationship are generally governed by fear. I usually find that the mother behaved passively towards a controlling father, resulting in fear of men rather than anger. The young girl makes a different interpretation of any abuse, which leads in later life to her seeking out what she feels are "safe" relationships with women.

I sometimes find that the home life was not at all negative or dysfunctional, but that a girl was treated as a tomboy and identified more with boys than girls. In later life, she may not see herself as a "girl" and may take a "male" job such as mechanic to prove to her family that she can be "the boy they always wanted" (see Case #60 in Chapter 14).

I have found that almost all women in lesbian relationships are in denial of the causes that turned them towards same sex relationships—be it anger or fear directed towards men—and that dislodging that deep-seated anger or fear can trigger a shift in consciousness that immediately snaps them into heterosexual relationships with few or no adjustment problems. Such clients quickly lose most of their lesbian friends, who may become hostile and abusive, seeing her as a "traitor."

The sudden shift apparently causes the women to question their own values, of which they may be in denial. As one would expect, those clients who have the hardest time adjusting are those who do not believe that such a shift is possible.

Returning to the issue of whether homosexuality is a "born in" trait, consider the client who has lived the majority of her past lives as man, and chose in this life to experience the female gender. However, it proved to be a difficult and uncomfortable adjustment. She found relationships with men to be too confrontational, so she chose to form relationships with women. However, sex as a woman turned her off, so she developed platonic relationships that worked for her.

Once she released all the misalignment on gender and made peace with her choice, she became adjusted and happy with who she was. She decided that any form of sexual experience was distasteful to her, so she became celibate. She could have gone through a sex change but decided she must have chosen the female gender for a reason and made peace with it.

Of course, some of my lesbian clients have successful, long-term relationships and have no desire to change. They have resolved their anger and fear, and clearly see the nature of their relationships.

In my seminars, I emphasize that you must face the choices you made before birth and work through the experiences your soul intended. You made these choices for reasons you may not understand in your Conscious Mind, yet they are before you now in the present time, and you must deal with the path you have chosen. It has been my experience that once you file the flight plan, there is little latitude to change it. If you had wanted a different path, you would have filed a different flight plan. Your intent in setting up this lifetime was to advance your evolution, and you had much help and wise counsel in making the best decisions for that.

The mistake many make is to assume that they have as good or better vision now than when they filed the plan. However, now that we are in physical bodies, our clarity is not nearly as acute, so we can be distracted by illusions and denials, which take us off the path. Most of the time, our ability to make life-changing decisions is so fogged up that we cannot make viable choices just to avoid rejection, pain, and suffering, let alone change our life path. Due to our childhood experiences, we get off the path and lose our direction. Of course, you can take any detour you want, even suicide, but it makes the journey longer.

A question that puzzled me was, "Why do we not see much AIDS or HIV in the lesbian community?" My research revealed a number of reasons: women are naturally more low-key in their sexual behavior, and seem to adjust more easily than men to a homosexual lifestyle. Also, despite the recent uproar about the sitcom star who "came out" on the show, there may also be less cultural bias against two women in a relationship than two men. Traditionally, when men have left home to fight wars, the women would often share households and care of the children, sleep in the same beds, and so on. Society appears to accept and accommodate lesbian women more than gay men because the former do not create a fanfare or are as visible. As a result, there is less stress from external rejection, and therefore, less internal self-recrimination, which is the cause of AIDS. (AIDS is a non-selective immune disorder, caused by total rejection of self.)

Homophobia is triggered in people who have fear and doubt about their own gender identity, traits often found among men in the fundamental religious community. Seldom are women vehemently homophobic. (The same reaction is often found in the pro-life movement, which appears to be controlled by conservative politically/religious men who want to deny women their rights.)

Gay men present a totally different picture. AIDS is rampant in the gay male community because many feel intense pressure from their own peers and may use their illness as a means of getting attention. While this works within their own community, for the most part, it elicits a negative reaction from the general population. This in turn causes self-rejection in the Body/Mind (see Chapters 7 through 9 for more information).

Contrary to popular belief, those who have a good relationship with self cannot contract HIV and AIDS. AIDS is not strictly a disease, but a breakdown in the immune system, leading to T-cell and the leukocyte blood counts so low that the body has no resistance to disease and invading organisms.

I have worked with countless gay male clients over the last 20 years, across the whole spectrum from the angry dominant to the passive. For some, their proclivity comes from past life experiences which again raises the question, "Are people born homosexual?"

My research has shown that, while a few are born with a particular gender in order to set up unfinished lessons, the real issue is *not* the gender one is born with. Almost invariably, regardless of someone's actual "plumbing," the basic programming that causes the choice for same versus different sex relationships stems from *childhood experiences*, and in particular, the relationship with the mother.

The main ingredient in the "personality recipe" is whether the mother was dominant and controlling, and whether the father was submissive or absent, i.e., no strong male model. We discovered that a strong, dominant, controlling mother, coupled with a passive, submissive or absent father caused many men to resent women and gravitate to a gay lifestyle. The cause is, however, not just the absence of a male role model. We might assume that single-mother families, with no male influence at all, would result in a higher proportion of gay men. However, the opposite turned out to be the case. *The key ingredient is the dominant mother.*

Without exception, all my gay male clients were rejected before they were born, many because the mother had wanted a girl and the father did not step in and support the son. Also, a son's past lives with the mother that have not yet been cleared are often the cause of subconscious anger, resentment or both.

Most of the time, a boy's conflict with his mother does not translate into good relationships with girls, or if he does get into intimate relationships as a teenager or young adult, he tends to choose girls or women who duplicate his mother's controlling behavior. In later chapters, we will see that the Body/Mind is a computer that is driven by its programs, and that it will drive a person away from what it perceives as painful or unhappy relationships by avoiding them. So, faced with choosing between aloneness and unhappy relationships with women, a man may well gravitate to the gay community.

Many of my male clients were "raised" as girls in their earlier years, some even being dressed by their mothers as girls until they entered school. This will definitely cause a gender identity crisis in teenage years. The mother of one of my clients actually introduced him as, "My son who should have been my daughter," and blamed God for making the wrong choice. A young boy brought up to think that God had made an error would obviously feel rejected by both his mother *and* God. So, he reasoned, how could any girl be his friend? He didn't make it too well in the gay community either, and was ready to commit suicide before he came to me as a client.

Many men in the gay community, I find, are angry, but overlay their anger with denial and act out obsessive/compulsive behavior. In 1990, a gay client was so impressed at the results I'd achieved with him and his friend in clearing their HIV status that he sponsored me giving a lecture in San Francisco to a group of gay men. We printed up flyers and booklets specifically aimed at our target audience, and I looked forward to making an impact on the gay community. Two days before the event, I was surprised when the owners of the venue backed out and refused us use of the hall. With no time to find a new location, we had to cancel the lecture.

My client remarked to me, "Most people do not believe that you helped me clear HIV. Because very few are really interested in healing themselves, I decided not to reschedule your lecture." In fact, he suffered such hostile backlash from his friends that he eventually left the gay community.

I am appalled at how few gay men are willing to entertain the idea of clearing HIV. We have achieved many miraculous healings, yet many HIV-positives are closed to the process (see chapter 14). Personally, if I was in a potential life-threatening situation, I would seek any help I could find, regardless of my opinion of the process. In my journey, I encountered many dead-ends, but at least I tried them. If you end up as a statistic in a death register, what have you accomplished?

On the other hand, with those clients who *are* willing to work out the original causes, we can make major changes. In some cases, when we release all the programs and sub-personalities driving the denial, they let go of the gay lifestyle and return to a "hetero" lifestyle with no desire to go back. The process of reintegration may take some time but they adjust very well.

I must reiterate that my intent is not to change people's lifestyles, but to foster peace, happiness, harmony, joy and unconditional love and acceptance in their lives. I see no need to suffer or exist in pain and conflict. What happens when we rewrite the programs and scripts is up to my clients. I have no agenda about what they should do with their newfound awareness. That is up to them. If they choose to stay where they are, fine. As long as they're happy doing it.

Bisexuals form a third group. These are experimenters who will engage in any form of sex that excites them. However, I have found that they are looking for a form of satisfaction which they seldom find. Their life seems to run on auto-pilot on every level. I have helped a few reclaim their personal power and take responsibility in their life so they can make a definitive choice in direction.

A fourth group is the *transgenders* or *trans-sexuals*. This gender maladjustment is described in psychiatry as dysphoria, or a desire to be physically the opposite gender. There are many causes for this gender identity situation; one seems to be genetic coding from past lives and the manner in which you were treated as a child. If you have lived many lives as women, you would have had many relationships with men. Suppose in your next (i.e., this) lifetime, you decided to explore life as a male, your life may or may not work depending on how you were treated by your parents and by your peers. Via pastlife bleedthrough, you may be more attracted to other men than to women, and even feel as though you should be in a woman's body. Your voice and secondary sexual features may hint at being a woman. This could put you in a difficult bind, which you may out-picture by playing the role of drag queen.

Most of these people feel that they are in a body of the "wrong" gender. They may not get along well with their peers because they feel they do not fit in nor are they accepted. As a result, low self-esteem can lead to intense self-rejection.

The challenge is that these people must validate themselves in order to be able to see through the veil of denial. With self-validation, your gender makes little or no difference to your self-image, and you can feel good about yourself without any withholds.

Many times, the flight plan has a built-in escape hatch in case the gender choice doesn't work out. Of course, this drastic step means surgical removal of the sex organs and other hormone-producing body parts.

We are not considering simply "playing" the role of the opposite gender, such as the drag queens who masquerade as women yet live as a male the other part of the time. There are men and women who carry on their daily work lives as one gender and switch to the other gender in social situations.

The mind is made up of four networked computers, and the stress on the Body/Mind system of the four minds being out of alignment could very well "crash" the system and lead to illness and disease. To escape the stress, one might ultimately seek hormone therapy or even surgery to complete the transgender switch. My experience with those who go all the way with a total sex change is that they end up better adjusted in their new gender. They tell me that it's not just about gender but about fitting in and feeling good about who they are. Unfortunately many early accounts about transgender change were lurid stories in the field of pornographic literature. However, this is changing as the respectable transgender community manages to pull away from past sensationalism, aided by psychologists and transition counselors. While such a major transition in lifestyle requires considerable support, it provides a new way of finding happiness for countless people.

I can personally identify with the transgender situation since my mother raised me as girl in my early years. I had two near-death experiences in an effort to escape my feelings of not fitting in, the first when I was only eight years old. My early programming and the way I felt about who I was caused me to delay going into puberty. In my early years, I gravitated to girls as playmates, but as I grew older, I engaged in more male activities. However, the other boys excluded me because I did not fit in. At age 12, I was only four foot ten, so they all towered over me, and would tease me, beat me up, and when I'd run away, they'd jeer and call me a sissy. Showering after gym was a nightmare because I had no body hair and the other boys teased me mercilessly.

From age 12, I was a closet cross-dresser. I admired and envied the attention the girls received, no matter what their height, but I kept my feelings strictly to myself. I had no idea who I was, except I yearned to be a girl because girls seemed to have a better time than I did. Of course, I realized that being a girl wasn't possible so I suppressed my feelings, resigned to living with simply not fitting in with either gender. All I wanted was to be a girl, and I couldn't understand why anyone would be attracted to boys. (None of the other kids ever called me homosexual because I just didn't have any obvious mannerisms.)

When I was 15, the Christine Jorgenson story became news. She was an army sergeant who went AWOL to Denmark for a total sex change. Because I was already deeply concerned about my gender identity, that story scared me.

When I was almost 18, I'd grew seven inches in a little over a year, was finally in puberty, and at last, other boys began to accept me. Girls already accepted me as a friend and buddy, but I was unsuccessful in attracting any into a relationship. At college, no one knew my past, and I readily attracted girlfriends. Once I found that my "male plumbing" worked, most of my longing to be a girl disappeared. At least, I assumed it had.

In the computers making up the Body/Mind, ignored programs do not conveniently "go away." They are still active even though we may suppress them into denial. In fact, mine went into denial of denial, so they didn't even exist as far as I knew. In 1985, however, I started on a spiritual journey to find myself, and by 1991, all those programs held in denial started spilling forth. All my desires about being a girl were still active and once more began to complicate my feelings about sex and who I was.

In 1995, I traded a session with a woman and to my surprise, all the hidden information started pouring out. "Talk this out and release it. Don't be shy about telling people about it," she advised. "You had a real tough time from thirteen to seventeen, didn't you."

As the files opened, she "saw" my cross-dressing and wanting to be a girl. "As far as I can see, you made the right decision for your path. You could have continued cross-dressing, had a sex change or become homosexual. You were really at the crossroads of your life."

I am still working out and releasing the programs and patterns from my past. I lived with these feelings and never told anyone how I felt, so I can understand how a transgender person feels because I have walked in their shoes for most of my life.

Harking back to the statement by Tara Singh: "You will not teach anything you have not experienced," it was an appropriate comment in my case. My earlier experiences helped me understand the sexual confusion many people face in their lives, and now that I've removed those files that were causing me problems, I'm looking forward to the remainder of my life being more productive.

So how do I feel about these concepts now? To me, life is a workshop. We come here for fun and soul evolution. Some people naturally have life handled; they say their lives work and I applaud them if that's true. (For success, you must be in contact with your true self, which most people are not because of subtle and insidious denial. Breaking through the denial usually takes an outside person. Even then, it is difficult because the mind is so clever in blocking programs.)

To me, life is a series of lessons. (If the word "lesson" irritates you, substitute which ever word you want, such as "experiences.") I know one thing for sure, however: When you file your pre-birth flight plan, you must follow your defined lesson plan. If a storm blows you off course, or if you decide you don't want to follow the plan you submitted, you can choose to rewrite it. However, if you want to add a few detours, you may not get to your desired destination in this lifetime, but that is free choice. If your detours result in a crash or you hit a storm, simply pick the pieces and head back out. When the storm is over, you may have to correct your vision, or forgive yourself for the detour, but your Higher Self and your Holographic Mind impose no time schedule on you. In fact, they don't care how many lifetimes your overall plan takes you.

A final note: When you recognize the illusion, you can leave denial behind and create a life of peace, happiness, harmony, joy, unconditional love, acceptance and financial abundance. If you do not have it now, then I hope the rest of this book provides you with some guidelines on how to get it. But that, too, is free choice. Have a great flight!

Chapter 3

Understanding the Theory of Healing

Before we begin, let's dispense with the term "spiritual healing." As one of my first teachers in the healing field described the process, "Until we clear the hurdle of our childhood emotional trauma and start building a foundation for our spiritual life, we can't even address the spiritual aspect of healing."

Too many people want to skip over the foundation-building and evolve to the spiritual aspect of their life path. Most people's denial of their own shortcomings will stop them from making the transition. Even though they may convince themselves that they are on the path of spiritual enlightenment, most people are deluding themselves because they have not dealt with basics of building a solid path to the spiritual realm. Many of my clients claim to be highly-enlightened spiritual beings, yet live in survival and illusion.

Most of this book deals with the basics of healing on the physical plane. Many people would like to believe that miracles come from the spiritual realm, yet we have proven this to be false. Over the last 18 years, I have worked with thousands of clients, many of whom didn't understand about enlightenment, yet once they committed to following my directions, miracle healing occurred. But we have to turn on our "God-switch" before miracles can take place. The presence of God is all of us, but most people's switches are turned off. Disease, illness or any form of lack is not a reality for a person who truly is on the spiritual path.

As we go through the dark nights of the soul, the dangers of the valley of the snakes, and wind our way around the obstacles in our path, we may get onto the spiritual path, but it takes time, intense discipline, commitment, and work. My book *Journey Into Light* details my interpretation and understanding of the process of spiritual healing as given to me from the spiritual realm. The spiritual path is a continuation of the path from the third-dimensional world, a process of separation from physical reality toward ascension and lightbody.

Healing is a process brought about by releasing the programs and core beliefs that drive our life. There is no disease, illness or dysfunctional behavior that just comes in and affects us by happenstance. Your mind controls every action you take and every situation that happens to you. Bacteria, viruses and fungi do not cause disease; they are the result of a breakdown in the body's immune system, again caused by the mind. We would like to blame our problems on someone else or "a disease going around" but it doesn't work that way. Growing up, my children were exposed to many contagious diseases but I would not allow them to be vaccinated for childhood diseases, yet they were never affected by any of them. Illness and disease are all caused by how you feel about yourself, and we set ourselves up for disease, illness and dysfunctional behavior.

We set everything up to get a certain payoff, usually without knowing how or why, or how to get out of the resulting situation. In fact, most of the time, we are so far into illusion that we cannot even understand why or how we ended up with our afflictions. Our first thought is that, "It is physical, I can feel the pain."

Pain is just a signal that something needs to be heard. It is also resistance to locating the cause. Your body is talking to you. But rather than listen to the message to locate the cause at the mental/ emotional level, we run to the doctor or take a drug to control the symptom. Anything that removes pain or discomfort without addressing the underlying cause is simply removing the charge and sidestepping the symptom. We will stop ourselves with strokes, heart attacks, cancer, MS, ALS, MSD and many other forms of illness and disease to either get someone to take care of us, or to get attention and love. Very few people recognize the base cause of the dysfunction; they are running away from themselves and the illusion that is driving their behavior.

The base cause is what happened in the beginning to cause you to react. It could have happened several thousands of years ago, or during childhood. How you respond or react to the catalyst governs how it affects you, and your interpretation sets up either a belief or a program. It may be many years before there is enough charge to cause an illness or a mental breakdown, but each time you run into the same catalyst, you will react based on the program or belief. Over time, programs and beliefs become patterns that cause you to react in the same manner each time.

The payoff for all illness and disease is the attention and approval you receive. Most of us will do anything to get attention, and are searching for someone who will provide the attention we crave. It may not be love, but that is how our mind interprets it. Children get sick to get attention. If they are getting enough love and acceptance, they do not get sick.

True love is acceptance without judgment. It is kindness and caring without any putdowns or attempts to control and manipulate. *Conditional love* comes in many forms, such as controlling a child's behavior with authority. It could be abuse at any level, even physical. Our viewpoint of love is based on how we interpreted our treatment in childhood. If as a child we were never picked up and hugged, or received no pats on the back, we grew up not knowing what approval is. As a result, we may have grown up without a basic unconditional love program. Without this program, people frequently get sick. Their life does not work yet they cannot find the cause. It is their body/mind trying to get someone, anyone, to give them attention.

Underlying any healing process is the ability to accept unconditional love. Most people are not able to accept love at a deep level of their being. Healing can only take place once we have released all the rejection and abandonment that we perceived throughout our life. We cannot receive approval and acceptance from others until we are able to give it to ourselves. As long as we feel others should give love to us, they will not do so in an unconditional manner. Many people seek out someone they can cling to in an effort to get attention, but almost everyone who offers support or help has a hook or a cord connected to it.

It is a basic human desire to have our existence recognized, and people will do anything to get recognition. Sickness is an obvious way of getting someone else to recognize that we are alive. Total rejection will cause death, because if you think you are not wanted, why be here? HIV and AIDS is a form of total self-rejection. Society does not accept you, so you reject yourself.

Most diseases are caused by selective immunity. AIDS is caused by total breakdown of the immune system, so there is no protection from disease. When the T-cell count drops to a level where the immune system cannot attack disease organisms, those organisms will flourish and overwhelm the body.

What then is the answer to the dilemma? Quite simply, the answer is unconditional love. It's that simple. It is the only answer that will heal the body permanently. To achieve this, we must remove all the programs, patterns and records from the Subconscious and Conscious Minds that are causes and precursors to disease and illness. The encrypted and encoded programs are the most damaging, because they were laid down before you were born. *In utero* programming recorded how your parents felt about this new child that they had created.

If you were rejected before you were born, you will interpret this input as "I am not all right. I am not acceptable." If your parents considered abortion or even just talked about it, this destroyed your self-esteem, self-worth, self-confidence and your validation of self. If you feel you have no value, you will continually choose people in your life who will confirm your worthlessness, and invalidate your credibility as a person. Bonding with your mother at birth is very important. Your earliest relationships with, and treatment from, your primary caregivers now control your life. How you interpreted the way people treated you set up childhood programming which in most people cause them to reject themselves.

The power of your mind is awesome. If the programs and beliefs are set up with an end result of rejecting the body, the mind will actually stop your body from assimilating drugs, herbs, minerals, vitamins, or any useful products.

The mind may allow selective acceptance if you make a commitment to taking care of your health. This is why many nutritional therapies work so well. They give the body adjuncts to help it clear the toxic materials that have been deposited, so it will begin to heal.

You can also use electronic instruments or acupuncture that will remove pain by allowing the body's electrical functions to return to normal. Many alternative therapies will help adjust the body through manipulation or energy transfer, but if you do not get to the base cause and remove the program, it will eventually cause the same condition to return.

When we review this information objectively without prejudice, we can see clearly that illness and disease are a state of mind. They exist in the body only because the beliefs, concepts, patterns and programs are driving them. In actuality, illness and disease do not exist. There are no contagious diseases, only contagious people who have programs, patterns, beliefs, interpretations and concepts about illness and disease that cause them to succumb to dysfunctional beliefs leading to physical breakdown.

I have proven beyond all doubt that allergies are beliefs with a causal factor (catalyst), that when activated, will flare up the allergy. Asthma works in the same way. We can blame some environmental agent, but that agent is tied to the core issue and base cause that created the allergy symptom in the first place.

I personally have not seen a doctor in over 25 years. I have been sick only once in the last 32 years, and that was because I worked 26 straight days without time off, while, at the same time, being under intense emotional release and extreme stress. Recovery took only a few days once I realized what I'd done to myself. Full healing took about two weeks because I'd stressed my body out to the point that my overworked adrenals had to recover.

The challenge is to be able to recognize the symptom and what your body is telling you. Few people can read their own "book" well, so the records are not accessible. Doctors will tell you, as they did me, you have no recourse, and the condition will continue to degenerate. A new challenge is that because your body/mind wants you to get the message, it builds up immunity to drugs, which nullifies their effect.

All we have to do is rewrite scripts by reprogramming the mind—simple when you have access to the records. If the script is coming out of a past life, you will have to release the karmic contracts and agreements you made with others in that lifetime. They follow you everywhere you go, from lifetime to lifetime. You cannot talk them out either; they have to be removed from cellular memory.

The script could stem from a belief you accepted which is not a reality. You constructed a situation out of an interpretation which is not even programmed in to your Subconscious mind, nor is it a body-based program. It exists only in your Middle Self's files. Such beliefs can be simply released with an affirmation.

To understand the theory of healing, you have to understand that nobody can heal you; you have to do it yourself. The "Catch-22" here is that first you must be willing to release yourself from the past programming without blame, guilt, justification, or judgment. Fear will drive you to control everything you contact. For example, if security is a major need in your life, this need will prevent healing. Another important factor for healing to occur is self-validation.

Many people believe that nutritional therapy promotes healing and sometimes it does. However, this still discounts the awesome power of the mind. If someone takes responsibility and commits to recovery, what they eat is *four times* more effective in healing compared with the person who follows a program because they were told it would work. It is the discipline and commitment that make the difference, not the food, herbs or supplements.

Many do, however, acknowledge the body component as the most important facet. You can rearrange the body fascia tissue and you can overwhelm and release a dysfunctional pattern, disease or illness with energy by laying of hands. That is true in part, but again, what is controlling the situation in the first place? The mind's computer may allow a situation to clear, but will it return when the same crisis becomes an issue again? If we view how the body heals itself, we find that it communicates using neuropeptides, chemicals that transmit electrical impulses which are picked up by the body's cells. Positive messages heal. Negative messages cause breakdown. We know that a scalar wave of 50,000 – 100,000 hertz is a standing energy wave that promotes healing. However, we do not know what the mind may do to block the energy. We have to go back to the programs and how they will effect the outcome of any process. Visualizations may work very well to recreate new programs, but the challenge remains to get the Middle Self to agree to work with you.

My books make statements such as, "You must take your power back. Reclaim your personal power. Take responsibility." To make a commitment and stick to it with discipline is hard for most people. They will confront the issues, then turn and run.

The most common problem in our society is the illusion, "My life is okay the way it is." Many clients have said to me, "I would like to change if it does not upset my life." This is a response fear-based reaction to change. Money and power also seem to be very important. "I can do it if it doesn't cost too much or cause financial difficulty."

People would rather stay in pain and illusion rather that confront the unknown. A client once called me after a session to say, "You really fouled my life up. It was a lot more comfortable before I had the session with you." We had opened a Pandora's box, and now she had to deal with some lessons and issues in her life which she did not want to confront. Her mother was also seeing me and had overcome some big obstacles in her life, so she assumed her daughter was ready to deal with her issues. Obviously she was not.

Other people tell me they feel better and their life is working better, yet they do not want to go any farther. Quite often, it's due to feeling better than ever before, and they can't see how it could be any better than it is now. When you reach a plateau where you have never felt this good before, you can think that this is all there is because you've never been here before.

With many clients, total change causes intense fear. Walking into uncharted waters can cause someone to retreat to what is known and safe. You do not have to be sick to step into wellness. Wellness is not sickness, but just the absence of dysfunctional programs that run your life.

Chapter 4

What Causes Illness, Disease and Behavior Dysfunction?

Medical researchers are right on track when they say that illness and disease are caused by a breakdown in the immune system. In a weakened immune system, T- cells, white blood cells and leukocytes do not have the numbers to attack viruses, bacteria and other invaders. At this point, the researchers get lost because they do not know how to boost the immune system. They think that antibiotic or other drugs can suppress viruses. This may happen, but many times the body's resources will refuse to work with drugs because the awesome power of the mind is able to neutralize their effect. The body/mind will heal itself if given the proper support, but the support is not drugs. The support is *LOVE.*

Most people are sedentary individuals who eat the "Great American Diet." Yes, it is important to eat right, since proper nutrition supports the body, but very few people know what proper diet is. It is also important when you eat various foods in your diet that you know where your vegetables come from. Most foods are devoid of minerals, so we need to supplement with minerals, but even with proper foods and supplements, you cannot heal your body. I have seen strict vegetarians with cancer, strokes and myriad other diseases. It is not what you eat; it is what is eating you *emotionally* that counts. For a full picture of proper diet and nutrition see my book *Being a Spiritual Being in A Physical Body.*

Eating properly takes commitment, discipline, consistency, and the ability to follow through. Clients have claimed to eat a good diet, but when I question their habits, what I hear is justification for why they fell into bad habits. I describe that as illusion and denial. Denial is not just an emotional problem. Nobody likes to have their bad habits pointed out, so most people will justify their behavior with excuses. It all comes down to commitment, discipline, and responsibility for yourself. Justification does not work. The only person you are fooling is yourself.

The human body has not changed or adjusted its dietary needs in millions of years. With a 32-foot intestinal digestive track, heavy protein such as red meat will putrefy before it passes through the intestines, and even then requires a pH of 2 (strong acid) to digest it. Then we wonder why we have an over-acid condition, which in turn causes ulcers and rheumatism. Normally, the intestine operates best at a pH of 5. Fish, nuts, beans and grains digest well in this medium. Fruits, melons and vegetables need no acid. If you mix fruit and protein in the same meal, you will create a winery in your stomach and it ferments because it takes different enzymes and acids to digest each one.

Sugar and white flour are poisons to the body. In fact, white flour products will turn to simple sugar in 30 – 60 seconds in your mouth.

The next ingredient is emotional well-being. Negative thoughts and feelings will break down your body faster than anything else. The emotions of fear and anger will cause more toxins in the body than a poor diet. My mother lived to 94 years with very few sick days. She was in the hospital only once—for elective surgery. Her saving grace was that she had good thoughts and forgave everybody. She ate a relatively good diet and did not drink or smoke, and her Christian Science background did not allow her to accept or believe in illness.

Most children get sick to receive attention, the payoff of almost all illness and disease. Life-threatening diseases are ways to escape from a situation or a conflict. Most stem from suppressing anger, or from fear of having to face some insurmountable situation or trauma. However, because our mind can make a mountain out of a molehill if it perceives something ahead that it does not want to deal with, the situation may be an illusion. We are talking about the mind's interpretation, not about someone's rational mind making a decision. When people cannot claim their power and take responsibility for their life, they will back out. In fact, rather than confront a controlling person, many people will set themselves up to contract a life-threatening disease. Usually these are codependent people who are unwilling to break the codependent bond and stand up for their views and desires. Rather than fight, they will back out of life.

Four of my clients chose death rather than stand up for themselves, and I gave them the last rites and offered them the opportunity to forgive themselves for taking their own life rather than face the issue.

We set up our life path by the time we are three years old, and few people are willing to break out of that mold and change. There are only two types of people: survivors and victims. Survivors will work against the programs, beating up their body because they will not give up. No situation will deter them. They will work through pain because they feel they don't have a choice. It must be done. Conversely, victims back out very easy, looking for someone to support them rather than push themselves. These are the people who die from life-threatening diseases.

Survivors will tend to put themselves in double-binds by working against the programs. They will use willpower to overcome dysfunctional patterns until the body finally breaks down because the Middle Self and Subconscious Mind will do anything to divert them from the path they have chosen. These minds assume that if you keep on the path you're on, you will be rejected, abandoned, or killed. This is unlikely, but your mind is not able to look beyond the current day. It is unable to see into the future, so it projects the past forward, assuming the past will be repeated.

In the case of past lives, your mind interprets the program created by the karmic contract or agreement, and acts as feels appropriate for your safety and survival. The fear may be unreal and ridiculous but it exists in your mind, so it sets up defenses against possible threat even though it may never happen. The mind evaluates situations as they come to you, and responds based on how it handled them in the past. If there are no programs to access, it will create one. The big IF here is: If *you* are directing your life, your mind does not have make a decision for you. *You* act on the sensory input and make the appropriate decision. If you have sold your power out to auto-pilot, then sub-personalities make your decisions for you, and they may not be the decisions you would make given the same input.

The major causes of most physical breakdowns are feeling rejected, not accepted, invalidated and abandoned. We all want to be accepted by everyone we meet, and will go out of our way to set up situations so that people will accept and validate us, many times subconsciously. Yet, the harder you try, the more you are rejected. Likewise, we do not intentionally mean to reject other people, but when we detect their need, it can feel as though an unwritten sign comes up saying, "Reject them, they are not getting the message or the lesson." It seems cruel at times, but that is how our Subconscious Mind works.

The awesome power of your mind will either heal you or cause you to get sick, and even die. Many times your mind causes illness without your conscious consent. If this happens, it is an auto-pilot response. If you do not clear the situation and find the base cause, it will continue until you give in and lose your will to live. At this point, it's too late to change the outcome. My father finally died of a lung congestion in the hospital after overcoming four life-threatening diseases, including pancreatic cancer. Once he made up his mind to give up, there was nothing we could do. He wanted to be near us and his grandson, but my mother would not move. She controlled him as she tried to do with me. Rather than take his power back and just move where he wanted to be, he chose death to escape the situation. Many years before that event, I made up my mind that I would not follow in my parents' path. Breaking out of that pattern was a major battle, because we generally follow our childhood model. Few people recognize the model they grew up with, so they continue in the same mold.

The major problem when dealing with physical/emotional breakdown is disciplining ourselves to face the issues that affect us. The more fear exists in our mind, the more we will resist acknowledging the very programs that are blocking recovery. Denial is the worst enemy of transformation, since it prevents us getting to the basic cause of the breakdown while creating a false sense of well-being.

During the winter of 1997, in a major breakthrough in the search for the cause for dysfunction, we located the sub-personality programs. My psychology training had taught Transactional Therapy, which focuses on the inner child, the critical parent, the inner adult and other sub-personalities which were assumed to be in the Subconscious Mind. Some researchers even advocated looking for disowned selves, or denied sub-personalities. In Voice Dialog, we talked with these disowned selves. (At least, we thought we were. Now that I have delved more deeply into the function of the mind, I am not so sure now with whom we were talking. I doubt that we were in contact with disowned selves all the time.)

Sub-personalities can run your life and appear very real. Chapter 6 describes how sub-personalities function and how to rewrite their scripts. Here, suffice to say that we must review what disease is. The medical field defines "disease" as: A malfunction in the body which causes an infection, a virus, bacterial growth, an abnormal growth of a cellular structure—in other words, anything they cannot control or understand.

Researchers give names to the syndromes they study. Then, they try to find drugs that control them. Or if surgery is possible, they will remove the offending part of the body without regard to the body's need for that organ or gland, on the assumption that if they remove the offending tumor or infected body part, the person is clear of the disease. While measures such as antibiotics and chemotherapy kill the offending body parts, they also kill all the body's other good anti-viral agents. This is all based on trying to kill the condition before they kill the patient.

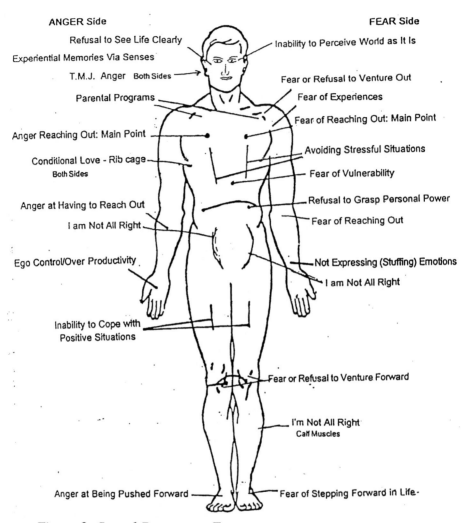

ANGER Side

Refusal to See Life Clearly

Experiential Memories Via Senses

T.M.J. Anger Both Sides

Parental Programs

Anger Reaching Out: Main Point

Conditional Love - Rib cage
Both Sides

Anger at Having to Reach Out

I am Not All Right

Ego Control/Over Productivity

Inability to Cope with
Positive Situations

Anger at Being Pushed Forward

FEAR Side

Inability to Perceive World as It Is

Fear or Refusal to Venture Out

Fear of Experiences

Fear of Reaching Out: Main Point

Avoiding Stressful Situations

Fear of Vulnerability

Refusal to Grasp Personal Power

Fear of Reaching Out

Not Expressing (Stuffing) Emotions

I am Not All Right

Fear or Refusal to Venture Forward

I'm Not All Right
Calf Muscles

Fear of Stepping Forward in Life

Figure 2: Stored Programs: Front

In the case of depression or emotional dysfunction, doctors use mind-altering drugs, which suppress one function and activates another. This treatment gives a false reading that can cause a reaction in the body/mind, and may or may not work.

Your body is an integrated unit. If you remove or suppress any part, the body will strive to regain balance, but that does not create wellness and heal the cause. My interpretation is: There is no such thing as illness or disease and I also believe there are no contagious diseases. Physical breakdown is caused by emotional

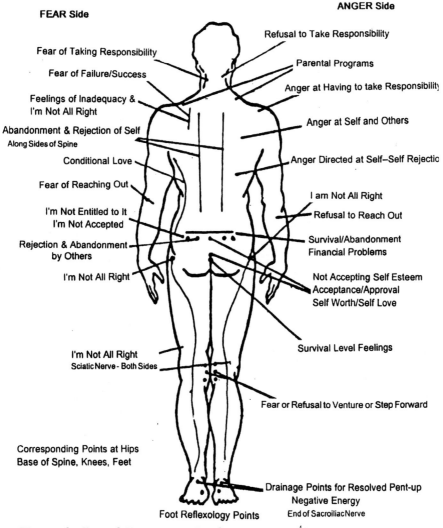

FEAR Side

ANGER Side

Refusal to Take Responsibility

Fear of Taking Responsibility

Parental Programs

Fear of Failure/Success

Anger at Having to take Responsibility

Feelings of Inadequacy &
I'm Not All Right

Anger at Self and Others

Abandonment & Rejection of Self
Along Sides of Spine

Conditional Love

Anger Directed at Self–Self Rejectic

Fear of Reaching Out

I am Not All Right

I'm Not Entitled to It
I'm Not Accepted

Refusal to Reach Out

Rejection & Abandonment
by Others

Survival/Abandonment
Financial Problems

I'm Not All Right

Not Accepting Self Esteem
Acceptance/Approval
Self Worth/Self Love

Survival Level Feelings

I'm Not All Right
Sciatic Nerve - Both Sides

Fear or Refusal to Venture or Step Forward

Corresponding Points at Hips
Base of Spine, Knees, Feet

Drainage Points for Resolved Pent-up
Negative Energy

Foot Reflexology Points   End of Sacroiliac Nerve

Figure 3: Stored Programs: Back

trauma, a dysfunctional program or a lesson coming up that needs
to be addressed. It is just a messenger. When we understand the
message it brings, we can clear and heal the illness or disease
immediately. The offending body part is only telling you that you
are rejecting it for some reason. Do we take it out because it is
malfunctioning?

Figures 2 and 3 indicate where in the body various programs
are stored.

The body/mind will reveal the cause so we can correct the programming. Once we find the cause and release the program and/or sub-personality driving the malfunction, it will recover its balance and heal itself. All we have to do is rewrite the script from which we are operating—a false belief or interpretation—or create a new program. Then we harness the body's own healing power, and when we operate from the new program, the body will heal itself perfectly.

This book repeatedly emphasizes that the mind creates diseases, illness and dysfunctional patterns and programs, a claim based on over 20 years of pragmatic evidence, documented in Chapter 14, Case Histories.

Chapter 5

How Body Cells Communicate

Many major speakers proclaim the effect of love on our Body/ Mind. Ten years ago, the medical community would have laughed at them, but today, even people from the medical field are making these claims. Medical researchers are now discovering that the body communicates positive or negative impulses to itself through chemicals such as neuropeptides (NP) and cytokinins.

For a long time, it was thought that only the brain released NPs, but now, we know that all cells communicate with NPs. NPs are like the acid in a car battery; turning the ignition on triggers a chemical reaction in the battery that is converted into electrical energy which cranks the engine. In our bodies, the NPs release minute electrical impulses that tell the various parts of the body what to do.

Our nervous system operates on electrical impulses, and messages of fear or anger create a destructive reaction in the body. The body cannot interpret this logically as, "Oops, this is a dysfunctional message." It does exactly what your mind instructs it to do. Our basic need is to receive love, so when we are in a loving state, the NPs transmit a love-based message, which heals the body. Illness, on the other hand, is lack of love.

The next time you hurt yourself and feel pain, try this experiment. Focus your mind on the location of the pain and surround it with love. Send love to the point of pain and feel the love releasing the pain. The pain will subside very quickly. Suppose you accidentally hit a fingernail with a hammer. Sending love to the nail will stop bleeding faster. It will not swell up or get black, and you will not lose the fingernail. I have done this myself many times over the years and I have suggested this process to many people. It works every time.

The main reason why researchers cannot find a cure for disease is that all disease is created by the mind's interaction with the body's cellular structure. You cannot remove a pattern from the mind by removing the dysfunctional part of the body. The dysfunctional program is still operating, and the illness will be created over and over, until the program is released. Conversely, a cathartic release cannot remove emotional pain. It may release the pent-up anger or fear energy, but it will not remove the program. If you do not release the program that caused the emotional pain, no amount of affirmations on forgiving and releasing a person will prevent recurrence. The program must be released from the physical body/mind.

Pain is an indicator of resistance; your mind is talking to you. All you need do is decipher the message and you can release the dysfunction. This is why Neuro/Cellular Repatterning works so well. We tell the Subconscious Mind to release, and the NPs do the work for us, provided that some program or sub-personality does not intervene to stop the process.

The Body/Mind is an amazingly sensitive bio-electromagnetic machine. Medical research has yet to understand that the body will heal itself if you release the dysfunctional programming and allow the original programs to perform as they were intended to do. When the limitations are removed, our cells can regenerate themselves from their original blueprints.

Medical research has discovered that cells communicate with each other using NPs, that the mind communicates through the endocrine system, and that it mobilizes the immune system. But doctors do not seem to understand the research findings. They are baffled by most diseases when drugs and surgery have only selective success. Admittedly, doctors do a great job in putting broken bones back together and patching up bodies that have been damaged in accidents, but when faced with a symptom that does not need repair, they are at a loss on how to handle the situation. Granted, doctors do achieve some success with disease, but their work does very little to isolate the condition causing the breakdown. However, people who want to be healed can do it very well themselves.

Medical research is stumped on another matter: why the same treatment used with two people with the same disease produces different results; one will die and the other recovers. It always comes back to the question, "Why? Why this selective immunity or selective remission?" However, when you understand the mind and how it functions, it is obvious that the programs are selective to a specific action.

Many books bear titles such as the *Cure for All Cancers*, and many others describe the cure for this condition or that condition. However, among those who have tried these processes, the success rate is not encouraging. Of course, some people successfully clear up a disease with the products and processes that are advocated, mainly because a belief is set up in their mind which becomes an inner "knowing." It is not actually the product or the process that heals them, but their commitment and belief. We are finally understanding the placebo effect in healing. Once they release the fear, their minds heal them. There are only two basic processes; healing which eliminates the syndrome permanently, and remission which puts the disease in limbo for a time.

I often work with clients on whom the medical profession has given up. They have been given a death warrant and told to get their affairs in order because they have only so many months to live, something that is communicated to every cell in the body. Some authority figure telling you, "You're going to die" just about wraps it up for most people.

Fortunately, some people have determination, and come to me. We reverse the disease syndrome and release the doctor's death warrant, all without drugs or surgery. Because all dysfunction is caused by fear, anger, self-rejection, invalidation, feeling unacceptable, not all right and lack of love, the only treatment needed is unconditional love. When this is transmitted, your body feels a sense of security and uses NPs to relay this love to your cells. They in turn release the disease or dysfunction and heal. Drugs and surgery simply cannot perform this miracle.

Chapter 6

Beliefs, and Cause and Effect

Our lives are run by beliefs, concepts, interpretations and attitudes that create programs. *In utero* interpretations that are recorded and locked into the cellular structure before we are born create beliefs which, if acted on, will become programs that control the balance of your life unless they are released. Apart from these, when we are born, there are no beliefs in our mind; they are all created from the time we enter physical life in a body.

Very seldom do we take any action that is not controlled by a belief, program or habit pattern. All beliefs are created by input to the data base—our thoughts and feelings, or other people's statements which we interpret. An authority figure can program your mind just by talking to you and explaining something. Anyone you accept as more knowledgeable than you on a subject becomes an authority figure to you, and your mind will accept their opinion as accurate, which then creates a belief. At this point, the belief can be transferred to a program if you react or feel threatened by the belief (see Figure 4).

Since your mind observes everything around you at all times, anything threatening to you can become a belief, too. Radio and TV will program your mind if you are not continually monitoring what your mind is taking in as sensory input. Subliminal advertising proves this point. About 30 years ago, just before the intermission in cinemas, researchers briefly flashed a message on the screen: "Buy popcorn now," and popcorn sales increased

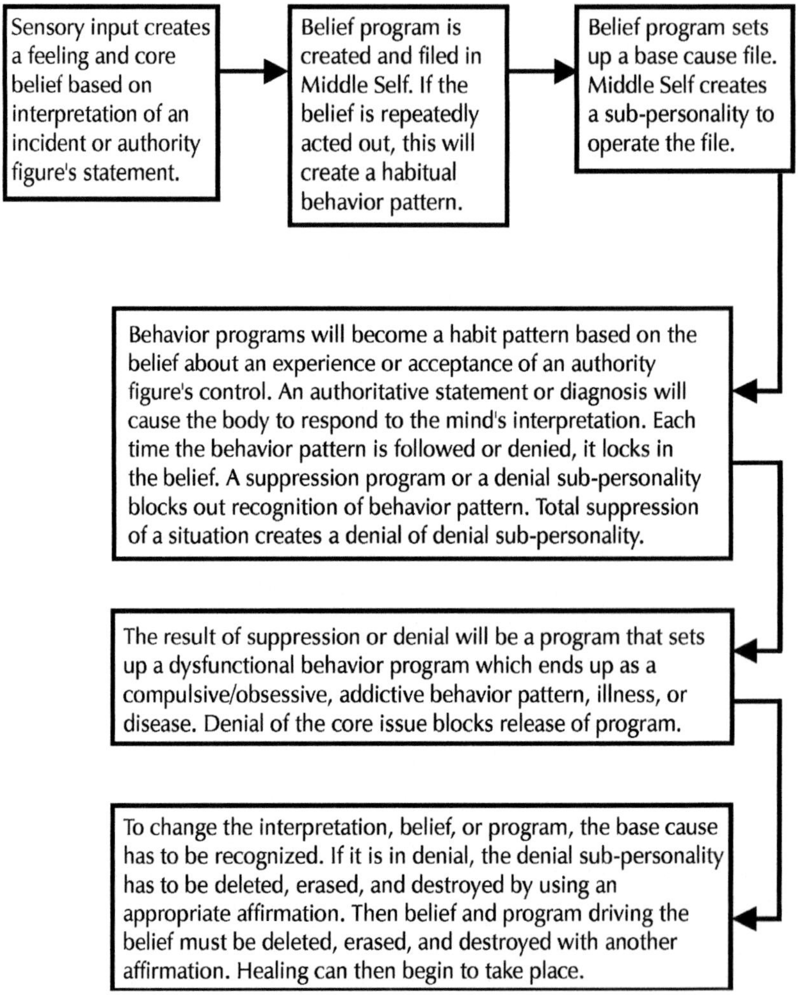

| Sensory input creates a feeling and core belief based on interpretation of an incident or authority figure's statement. | Belief program is created and filed in Middle Self. If the belief is repeatedly acted out, this will create a habitual behavior pattern. | Belief program sets up a base cause file. Middle Self creates a sub-personality to operate the file. |

Behavior programs will become a habit pattern based on the belief about an experience or acceptance of an authority figure's control. An authoritative statement or diagnosis will cause the body to respond to the mind's interpretation. Each time the behavior pattern is followed or denied, it locks in the belief. A suppression program or a denial sub-personality blocks out recognition of behavior pattern. Total suppression of a situation creates a denial of denial sub-personality.

The result of suppression or denial will be a program that sets up a dysfunctional behavior program which ends up as a compulsive/obsessive, addictive behavior pattern, illness, or disease. Denial of the core issue blocks release of program.

To change the interpretation, belief, or program, the base cause has to be recognized. If it is in denial, the denial sub-personality has to be deleted, erased, and destroyed by using an appropriate affirmation. Then belief and program driving the belief must be deleted, erased, and destroyed with another affirmation. Healing can then begin to take place.

Figure 4: How a Belief Is Created

by 150 percent. The message was not detectable by the audience, but since most people's Conscious Mind operates on auto-pilot, the message was taken in, recorded and acted upon.

When we are children, our parents set up much of our belief system by the way they care for and treat us. Conversations that we overhear that have no basic inference to our life can set up beliefs that will play out later in life. Childhood events can make serious imprints on our mind.

One of the most troubling cultural myths that has no truth concerns hereditary dysfunction, illness or diseases that are carried from generation to generation. It is the *belief* that is passed on to the children by the parents, not the *condition*. In work with countless clients, we have released the whole disease syndrome by affirmations acknowledging the situation and forgiving the person from whom they accepted the erroneous belief.

A belief will become a program if it is in the file long enough for it to become a habit pattern. If the habit pattern becomes strong enough to create a program, then a Middle Self sub-personality will adopt the program and lock it in. If we have sold our power out to the Middle Self and are on auto-pilot, this will also create a sub-personality in our Conscious Mind. If we do not want to deal with the experience or the trauma, we will bury it with a denial.

If we choose to forget it and avoid it totally, we put it into a "denial of denial" sub-personality. Most of this programming is done without our conscious knowledge. The more we rely on our survival self, the further we go on auto-pilot. As a result, more feelings, emotions, beliefs and programs get suppressed and buried to the point that we end up denying that a program or pattern exists.

We interpret all sensory input. If the input is a feeling, you understand its context, and it does not threaten you, then you will address it and let it go. However, if you feel threatened, say by a large dog, your interpretation can create a belief (that dogs are dangerous). If the feeling is one involving rejection or being criticized (say by your parents for putting yourself in harm's way), it will trigger an emotion and you will react according to the belief you have about that feeling (say, that you are dumb for doing it). If at the time of the incident, a catalyst is present (say, the dog's barking), it will be recorded as threat. Every time the catalyst situation arises (you hear a dog bark), you will react as if the whole incident will happen again. As a result, the catalyst will trigger an illness such as having an asthma attack in the presence of a dog.

One of my clients had a severe allergy to the goldenrod flower. I couldn't understand why until we found that her mother had chased her around her backyard and repeatedly beat her up in an angry rage. The goldenrod came into the belief because it had been in full bloom during that episode.

With many of my clients, a doctor has diagnosed an illness, and then the illness has turned into a disease. When a belief is driving an illness, there seems to be no way out. Ultimately, a belief can actually kill a person if it is imbedded in the mind and the person cannot see a way out. In cases like this, medicine has no way of stopping the disease.

A friend who is also a nurse told me a baffling story. She was providing home care for housebound patients who didn't need to be hospitalized. One patient was getting increasingly weak, and could no longer get out of bed. Finally he was unable to write or hold anything. The doctor hospitalized him for tests to determine what to do, but after a battery of tests, concluded there was nothing wrong with his body except it was deteriorating, and the patient just wanted to die. On being told that her husband was dying, his wife got sick, too, and died within a month. To my friend's amazement, the day his wife died, he started recovering and, within a week, walked out of the hospital totally healed. Neither she nor the doctor could explain the situation.

How could this happen, my friend asked. This was not a miracle, since there was no life-threatening illness or accident to recover from. No one facilitated his healing because the nurses had given him up for dead. The answer was that he was trying to escape his wife's covert control and codependency, and the only way he could find was to die. She had controlled his life to the extent that he wanted to escape. She had so much control over him he could not leave her physically so he chose this method. His belief was that he could not escape his wife and her control, so he was backing out of life.

With her husband's death imminent, the wife no longer could control him, so she became frustrated and died. Then, since his wife could no longer control him, he decided to come back to life and pick up his life again, with no ill effects from the ordeal.

Oddly, he was unable to communicate with anybody at the time, and no one had told him about his wife's death, so how did he know she was dead? Our mind does not just work in a linear time-frame on the physical level only. It has amazing abilities to access information that we don't think we have available to us. The nurses reported that he started to become more aware and awake right around the time his wife passed over. He had been close to death, yet somehow he got the message that he was now free of the cause of his impending death and walked back into life. (This also happened to my father but he did not get the message that he had to reclaim his personal power and take responsibility.)

An obvious question is, if the belief is somehow erased, does recovery happen every time? I have found the answer to be yes, it works every time, if you can erase the belief and concept. If you are doubtful or skeptical, then it will not work. This, too, must be released.

I have cleared the causes and the core issues with many clients, yet the dysfunction remains. Why is this? You can believe what we're doing at a conscious level, but all four minds must be in agreement and aligned with the goal. The next step has to be a *knowing*—not just belief or faith—to cause the final healing to happen. Both belief and faith are fear-based, as you are assuming something only *might* happen. If it fails, then you can blame the process or the practitioner. In other words, you're hedging your bets. The real cause is doubt and fear. It is an inside job. No one creates your reality for you; you do it all. For any path or addiction you choose, all we need do is find the belief that's driving it.

A client once asked me if we could determine whether her husband and son died from a belief. We accessed their karmic records and found out the cause of death—a belief in hereditary heart disease. According to the medical doctors, they were deemed incurable because there really was no disease, but they both died from the belief that they had inherited it.

Beliefs can be passed on to a person or a group, and if enough people accept a belief, it will become a reality for the group. One of the more bizarre beliefs I run into is that our chakras have a "mind" and can think rational thoughts. My understanding is that chakras are non-physical energy centers, connected to the various endocrine glands and organs, and located in the mental and emotional energy fields. They do pick up and transmit feelings, and put them out as an energy that has to be interpreted. That the heart chakra can make rational decisions is a myth, yet many people believe it. To say, "My heart is not in it" is a figure of speech, not a reality. All you are really saying is that you do not want to participate in something. That is a conscious decision or a programmed response from a belief (or a sub-personality if you are on autopilot).

Clients tell me they have a block in their throat or fifth chakra. How can this happen? It starts with a belief and a feeling, which is transferred to the emotional field. If we react to the feeling, then it will appear in the body as, say, a sore throat. To deal with it, we must listen to what the body is telling us. If we get the lesson or action we have to take, the sore throat will disappear.

Harold Saxon Burr, an English researcher in the 1930s, found what he called "L fields" (aka, the auric or energy field). By using his clairvoyant/clairaudient abilities to get the message before it appeared in the body, he found that he could diagnose illness and disease up to two weeks before it actually manifested in the body. The body talks at many different levels; the challenge is to decipher the message.

In summary, mind control is more prevalent then ever before. At every level of our society, we are bombarded by controlling messages, and must be vigilant about all sensory input coming to us, as our mind records everything that it picks up. We must detect and cancel all information that does not support our life path. The best way to this is to be observant and, when we encounter something we don't want to take in, say to ourselves, "Cancel."

People may inadvertently say things to us that they do not realize will cause harm, so do not blame them. We should be especially wary of authority figures. Anyone can be an authority figure if your mind so defines them, such as when someone knows more about a subject that you do. We must also eliminate and remove all the autopilot sub-personalities that are driven by the need to control, manipulate, or blame, or by anger and fear beliefs, programs and habit patterns.

Chapter 7

How the Mind Functions

The awesome power of the mind can run your life without your consent, since it operates very effectively without your input. Therefore, understanding how it functions is critical. In fact, the most important part of any therapy or healing process is understanding how the mind functions. Earlier chapters have skimmed this subject, and this chapter examines what we have found in 20 years of research.

Historically, what we thought of as "ego" is totally off-base. Discovery that the Ego was not the controlling factor in our mind was a major shift in my healing philosophy and the concept of how the mind functions. Until 1992, I was after Ego because the traditional belief in psychology and in many cultures painted it as the enemy in our mind. I had followed *A Course In Miracles* since 1977 so, for me, Ego was the formidable driving force that kept us separate from God and ourselves. This all changed in 1993 when I found that we were up against a saboteur that we could not control. With the help of the practitioners I was training, we spent a considerable amount of time working on what this driving force in the mind was that seemed to control our behavior. What we found was mind-blowing to say the least. It was not Ego at all. Ego had nothing to do with control nor did it want to control any part of us. It is just the file manager for our Subconscious Mind. Ego *per se* does not run our life; it is only the secretary, librarian and memory retrieval system. The conventional concept of it as "the enemy" is totally false. Of course, if you beat it up, it will defend itself but, if you make friends with it, it will serve you well.

There really is no "enemy" in our mind, even though it seems at times that our mind is working against us. The closest part of our mind that could be described as an "enemy" is our controller sub-personalities—manipulator, judger, authority, self-righteous, justifier and critical parent. They can act in what we call ego-like habit patterns, and we must accept that *we* have allowed all the programs, habit patterns and sub-personalities to be programmed in to our mind. *That we created it all can be a hard pill to swallow.*

Life is like a crossword puzzle in which the blacked out squares are karma that we must take care of at some point. The open squares represent free choice in which *we do only what we want to do, no matter how we made the decision. We have a choice every minute of each day to take responsibility.*

The Middle Self

The concept of middle self has been in the Hawaiian culture for thousands of years but the missionaries suppressed native philosophy and concepts about the mind, so they are not generally known or accepted by Western psychology. It has taken me almost ten years to prove that my concept of the Middle Self's sub-personalities are the controllers, and not Ego. Most circles are unaware of how these sub-personalities function so they hold onto the old Ego concept. Ego is nothing more than an operating system in our Subconscious Mind. It can be reprogrammed very easy (see affirmation in Chapter 15, Practice of N/CR).

Few people are aware that, every minute of every day, their mind has an ongoing dialogue with itself. As the previous day's sensory input is filed away, it accesses related data in the files in your Subconscious Mind. It never sleeps; it is on duty 24/7.

In my research, I ran into a barrier to getting all the programs cleared. We would release all the programs the Subconscious Mind was holding on a particular emotional pattern, get Ego into alignment, and reach consensus with the Conscious Mind's intentions, yet we were not getting a total release. The situation would resurface or create a new set of breakdowns. We finally discovered the source of the conflict: Middle Self.

Middle Self consists of (see Figure 5):

- *Conscious Rational Mind*, the functional aspect, the "keyboard" where you, the conscious self, program and control your life.
- *Autopilot*, which can run your life without your control through its Justifier and Judgment subpersonalities. When people go on auto-pilot, they give their power away to a another subpersonality that they

HIGH SELF
Connection to GOD Self. Akashic Record Telephone operator Connection to Source Mind and the Hall of Records

MIDDLE SELF
Conscious Rational Decision Making Mind Auto Pilot (Justifier, Judger sub-personalities) Inner Middle Self (Control, Manipulator sub-personalities) Instinctual Self, Survival Self

LOWER SELF
Subconscious Mind Ego Holographic Mind (Soul Mind)

Figure 5: The Middle Self

created to escape from some situation or experience. Middle Self sub-personalities can set up auto-pilot operating systems in the Conscious Rational Mind and, as a result, run our lives without our consent or control.

- *Inner Middle Self*, with its Control and Manipulator subpersonalities.
- *Survival Self/Instinctual Mind,* which operates out of the limbic part of the brain Some people describe it as the animal or reptilian mind. Brain researchers theorize that this is the oldest part of the brain. I feel this could be inaccurate since its actions interleave with the actions of the Inner Middle Self, which operates from beliefs, concepts, interpretations and attitudes. These, if acted on for a period of time, will create programs and patterns. It also has a set of sub-personalities for each concept or belief.

The committee in your Middle Self is also in session 24 hours a day. It doesn't care if you listen in, since it feels that it operates quite well without you. If you are not making the decisions that affect you and are not taking responsibility for what happens in your life, your sub-personalities will make the decisions for you. They may not make the choices you would consciously make, but someone has to be at the helm all the time.

Auto-pilot may do a fine job of guiding you through your day if there are no crises or confrontations where you have to make decisions, but if a situation occurs that requires decisive action, someone has to make that decision. If you are not at the helm, your Inner Middle Self's irrational mind, your auto-pilot, and its committee will make your decisions for you.

Middle Self bases its action on how you have handled the situation in the past. It scans the files and, if no program exists, the committee will take whatever action best promotes its survival. If you are in a situation that, at a conscious level, you consider beneficial to you, but which your committee of sub-personalities views as threatening, it will try to sabotage you.

If you are not in total control of your life, your Middle Self committee will try to stop any threat to its power. If you give it the message that you are claiming your personal power and taking responsibility for your life, it will readily relinquish its power to you. However, at first, it won't trust you, and you will have to prove yourself.

To harness the awesome power of the mind, we must control it. This power is available on demand, but first you must get your committee aligned with your goals and purposes, otherwise it will sabotage you. If, in the past, you have given it free reign or sold out your power to it, you must reclaim it.

The first task is to make friends with your Conscious Rational Mind and your Middle Self and its sub-personality committees. Next, you give them a structured format with parameters to follow, and most of the time, you can get them to work with you. The more you have separated yourself from controlling your life (say, by being a victim), the longer the path to reclaim control of your world.

There is a payoff in each path we take, usually in the form of getting attention or a substitute for love. We all want to be loved, validated and accepted, and the number one priority of your Middle Self subcommittee is the need to be validated and loved. It therefore views any concentrated form of attention as love, whether it is physical or emotional kindness and caring or abuse. It will accept anything as a substitute for love, other than outright rejection. The actual form does not seem to matter as long as other people acknowledge that we make a difference in their lives. Depending on its interpretation of the available options, Middle Self may choose victim or survivor.

To people who have been abused, this analysis may seem callous. Yet unless they accept that they set up the abusive situation based on the lessons they needed to learn, and that they perpetuate the situation until they "get" the lesson, it will continue to control their lives. To come to this point, they must recognize that when they reclaim their personal power and stop blaming others for their plight, they can pull out of victim consciousness. The final lesson is to love and forgive those who abused them. It is very hard to accept that you have to forgive those who hurt you, but the lesson is not released until you do.

The main challenge is to understand how your mind operates. Your Subconscious Mind is simply a computer that makes no rational decisions, and cannot "think out" situations. What we call the autonomic nervous system is actually a set of indigenous programs in the Subconscious Mind that automatically controls organs, the endocrine system, and the cellular functions of the body. It uses programming already in the files to tell all the cellular computers how to control the body's organs and endocrine system. Because it controls your endocrine and immune systems functions, in effect, your mind controls your resistance to disease.

Most of the mind's inner dialogue goes on without our conscious recognition, yet is faithfully stored in your computer's files. Now, any sensory input can compromise the function of the original program, and if sensory input or emotional trauma overloads a file, your body starts talking to you through little pains which, if you don't listen, can grow into a more serious dysfunction. The first message may be just a whisper. The next one will be a pain or a malfunction such as an illness. If you do not get that one, the next may be a more serious knock on your door, up to and including a life-threatening disease. Most people do not see this progression creeping up on them, and generate a landslide of business for doctors, who try to treat the symptom. Unfortunately, the symptom has nothing at all to do with the computer program or the action of the sub-personality responsible.

Traditionally, we used to assume that "self-talk" was Ego and Subconscious Mind carrying on an internal discourse or making observations and judgments about the outside world. I see now that the Middle Self's sub-personalities are in constant dialogue, which includes accessing information from the Subconscious Mind's database. (They request information from Ego, but Ego is very seldom in on the dialogue.)

When we see how the mind operates, we become aware of the awesome power of the mind to run and control our lives. For optimum functioning, we must get all sections of our mind into alignment. When we get Middle Self and Lower Self to integrate with Higher Self, we can really make progress.

The Operation of the Mind

As Figure 6 shows, the process begins with receipt of sensory input, be it a sound, sight, smell or touch. However, the stimulus can also be a thought or memory.

1. **Sensory input** (visual, auditory, physical feeling, meta-communication, and information from higher sources). and **new thought forms** (creative, inventive and intuitive), plus **processing dialogue** (negative or positive thought forms, flash back, memories, misinterpretations) are fed to the Middle Self.

2. **Middle Self interprets** the perceived information, processing through the Conscious Rational Mind or autopilot sub-personalities. (Search for programs of past reactions or responses, and the Reaction/Response is controlled by the operational program in the Middle Self and

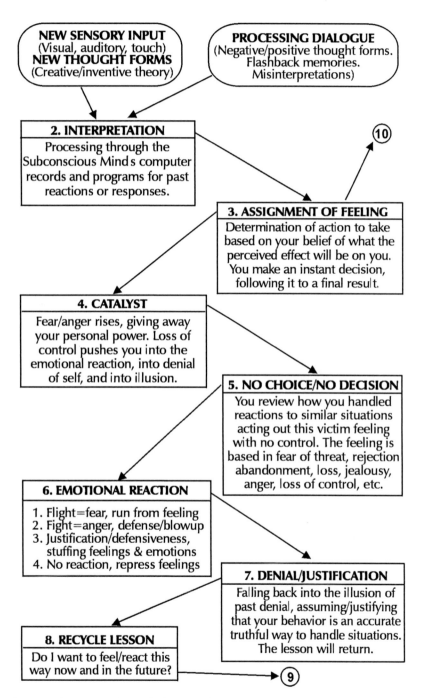

NEW SENSORY INPUT
(Visual, auditory, touch)
NEW THOUGHT FORMS
(Creative/inventive theory)

PROCESSING DIALOGUE
(Negative/positive thought forms.
Flashback memories.
Misinterpretations)

2. INTERPRETATION
Processing through the
Subconscious Mind s computer
records and programs for past
reactions or responses.

⑩

3. ASSIGNMENT OF FEELING
Determination of action to take
based on your belief of what the
perceived effect will be on you.
You make an instant decision,
following it to a final result.

4. CATALYST
Fear/anger rises, giving away
your personal power. Loss of
control pushes you into the
emotional reaction, into denial
of self, and into illusion.

5. NO CHOICE/NO DECISION
You review how you handled
reactions to similar situations
acting out this victim feeling
with no control. The feeling is
based in fear of threat, rejection
abandonment, loss, jealousy,
anger, loss of control, etc.

6. EMOTIONAL REACTION
1. Flight=fear, run from feeling
2. Fight=anger, defense/blowup
3. Justification/defensiveness,
   stuffing feelings & emotions
4. No reaction, repress feelings

7. DENIAL/JUSTIFICATION
Falling back into the illusion of
past denial, assuming/justifying
that your behavior is an accurate
truthful way to handle situations.
The lesson will return.

8. RECYCLE LESSON
Do I want to feel/react this
way now and in the future?

⑨

Figure 6: Operation of the Mind

Subconscious Mind.)

3. **Assignment of feeling:** Determines what action to take. At this point, you have two choices: Reaction or Response. Your choice is based on past belief or perceived effect from installed programs.

4. **Catalyst:** Loss of control pushes into fear/anger, degenerating into emotional reaction and giving away personal power.

5. An **Unconscious Decision** is made in an instant based on Catalyst as to the action to take—flight or flight.

6. **Emotional Reaction:** No choice/ no decision, result:
   a. Flight/avoidance. Run away from feeling;
   b. Fight/confront. Defensive, blowup out of control;
   c. Defense of action. Justification of action, denial feelings;
   d. No reaction, total avoidance with repression of feeling/emotion;
   e. Either go into denial or wake up to the lesson and review the situation that caused the reaction.

7. **Denial/Justification:** Falling back into the illusion of the past denial as a victim, justifying behavior as the only responsible reaction we could take. At this point illusion and denial may form a denial-of-denial sub-personality, If this happens, the cause of the behavior is totally suppressed *as if it does not exist.* We assume that our reaction was an accurate truthful way to handle the situation.

8. **Recycle Lesson:** At this point, you may review your behavior and ask yourself, "Do I want to feel/react this way now and in the future?" If you can do this, you can recycle the lesson.

9. **Recognition of Denial:**
   a. Review behavior you deem as ineffective.
   b. Recognize the effect of the lesson.
   c. Move into recovery and erase the ineffective program and remove the sub-personality driving the program.
   d. Remove denial-of-denial sub-personalities if you can recognize them

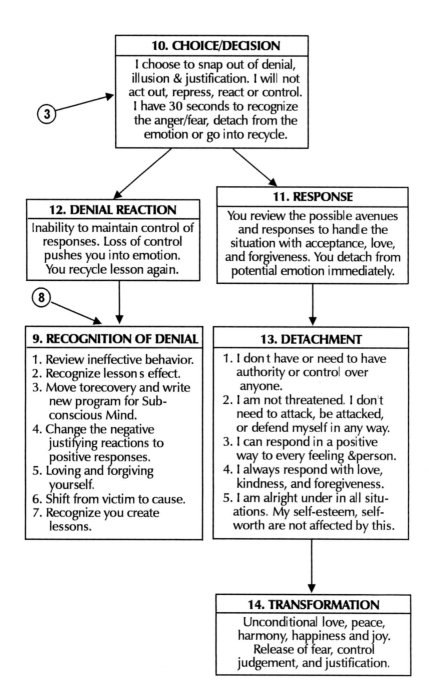

10. CHOICE/DECISION

I choose to snap out of denial, illusion & justification. I will not act out, repress, react or control. I have 30 seconds to recognize the anger/fear, detach from the emotion or go into recycle.

(3)

12. DENIAL REACTION

Inability to maintain control of responses. Loss of control pushes you into emotion. You recycle lesson again.

(8)

11. RESPONSE

You review the possible avenues and responses to handle the situation with acceptance, love, and forgiveness. You detach from potential emotion immediately.

9. RECOGNITION OF DENIAL

1. Review ineffective behavior.
2. Recognize lesson s effect.
3. Move to recovery and write new program for Sub- conscious Mind.
4. Change the negative justifying reactions to positive responses.
5. Loving and forgiving yourself.
6. Shift from victim to cause.
7. Recognize you create lessons.

13. DETACHMENT

1. I don t have or need to have authority or control over anyone.
2. I am not threatened. I don't need to attack, be attacked, or defend myself in any way.
3. I can respond in a positive way to every feeling &person.
4. I always respond with love, kindness, and foregiveness.
5. I am alright under in all situ- ations. My self-esteem, self- worth are not affected by this.

14. TRANSFORMATION

Unconditional love, peace, harmony, happiness and joy. Release of fear, control judgement, and justification.

    e. Change the negative justifying reactions to positive responses.

    f. Rewrite a new program and install it in the files.

    g. Recognize that you create all lessons, so that you can shift from victim to cause.

    h. Love and forgive yourself for allowing this to happen.

10. **Choice/Decision:** When we recognize this decision point, we have about 30 seconds to detach from the emotion and respond in an effective way. State, "I choose to step out of denial, illusion and justification. I will not act out, repress, justify, manipulate, try to control or judge another's behavior."

11. **Response:** If we are not able to detach from the emotion immediately, we will go into recycle. If we can respond effectively and positively, we review the possible avenues and responses to handle the situation with acceptance, forgiveness and unconditional love. At this point we were able to detach from the emotion and avoid separation from self.

12. **Denial Reaction** will take over due to our inability to maintain and control our response, Loss of control will push us into the emotion. We recycle the lesson again.

13. **Detachment:** Hallmarks of successful detachment are the ability to recognize the feeling with a new viewpoint and interpretation, and honestly say to ourselves:

    a. This is not an attack on myself worth or who I am.

    b. I don't have or need authority or control over anybody.

    c. I don't need to attack, be attacked or defend myself since I am not threatened unless I believe it can happen.

    d. I can respond in a positive manner to every feeling or situation and all people at all times.

    e. I am alright under all conditions, in all circumstances, in all situations at all times.

    f. My self-esteem and self-worth are not affected by this experience.

g. I can respond with love, kindness and forgiveness at all times.

14. **Transformation:** When we are able to recognize that we do not need control or authority at any time. We will not be attacked at any time, nor do we have to defend ourselves or attack back, When we release fear, anger, control, authority, judgement and justification, we have made it through the transfiguration, and unconditional love, peace, happiness, harmony and joy is our entitlement.

Split Personalities

Sub-personalities are the driving force behind habit patterns. If you follow a certain action, belief or interpretation long enough, it will become a habit pattern. If you deny that you are following that pattern, it will become a denial sub-personality. If you persistently deny the program that the pattern created, you may become totally separated from yourself and move into denial of denial. If you disassociate from yourself at times of great stress, you become a split or multiple personality. At this point, the sub-personalities become who you are, as you become totally separated from self.

Most people with this dysfunction are labeled as psychotic or schizophrenic, a condition in which it is easy for a possessive spirit being to walk in and take over. This is usually the end result. At this point, people can leave for short times (a few minutes to hours), but sometimes, people leave for many years, with no recollection of what they have done or where they have been. This demonstrates the awesome power of the mind to operate without our approval or direction.

All mental dysfunction is caused by a choice by the mind to create another world to run away from some traumatic experience. Almost all dysfunction of this type starts with a childhood experience. The child will escape into an imaginary world that he or she sets up to avoid pain. I refer to this as "escaping into the Magical Child," which is controlled by the Inner Child sub-personality. This will be carried through life until it released.

I have worked with many people who "disappear" in a sense. They are physically in the same body but they lose track of time. When they get back in their body they cannot account for days, and sometimes months or years. If we can unwind the programs and experiences, we can bring the original personality back.

People can also disappear when they go on auto-pilot and give their power away to another created sub-personality that was created to escape from some situation or experience. Middle Self sub-personalities can set up auto-pilot operating systems in the Conscious Rational Mind and as a result, our life is run without our consent or control.

Figure 7 portrays the formation of a split personality:

1. Sensory input from a trauma, pain, situation or any form of abuse will cause a person to escape into a magical child.
2. Middle Self creates a sub-personality to accommodate the escape.
3. Person goes on auto-pilot or has been on auto-pilot at times, This evolves into multiple sub-personalities that control the mind function. The person shuts down and the original personality self shuts down. Split personalities are a series of sub-personalities running a person life.
4. Multiple personality disorder and Schizophrenia are generally caused by an attached spirit being who takes over becoming another personality self.

Sometimes I have been able to pull clients back and remove all the attached beings if they want to do so, but often, they have made the choice to die and do not want to come back. I have found sometimes that they are angry, and force other people to take care of them.

Parental Legacy

In well-balanced people, the levels of the mind are tightly integrated, but they may operate separately due to separation in childhood. Few people have parents who direct and support their

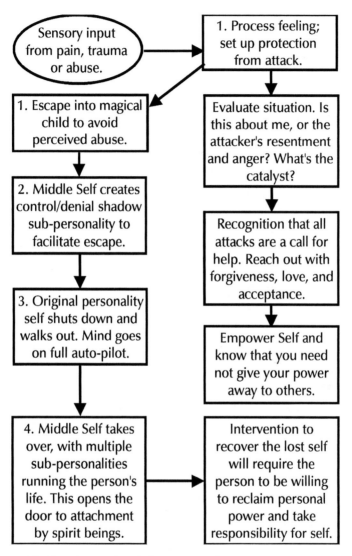

Figure 7: Creation of a Split Personality

children to become creative thinkers and support the development of their self-esteem and self-worth. Self-confidence comes from proper direction, which gives a child the feeling of making the right decisions. Most children do not feel they are alright and acceptable, so they reject themselves and do not have confidence in their actions. Parents unwittingly program their children for failure by being critical and putting them down.

Most of the time, parents are not aware of their own programs that cause them to compete with their children and make them feel they can never match up to the parents' desires. The biggest villains in this behavior pattern are the controller and manipulator sub-personalities—everything has to be done their way or it's not acceptable.

Lower Self has its agenda to keep you on track, yet it cannot make decisions or influence your behavior. I used to believe that Ego ran our life when we did not take control, but it does not have that power at all, although blaming it is a popular pastime.

Middle Self will buy into Ego's culpability because it takes the heat off its own activities. Middle Self creates individual selves (sub-personalities), that it uses to create more separation and fragmentation.

If you were abused by a parent or a partner, you can choose to hold onto the anger, fear and self-rejection. Alternatively, you can face the denial and illusion, and then let it go. Are there any tools in your life that will help you to release the illusion and open the door to peace, happiness, harmony, and joy with financial abundance and unconditional love? Have you tried them and do they work? *The challenge is to recognize the lesson, that no one can hurt you; only you can.*

Following a traumatic situation, what causes you to feel emotions about the trauma? It is your interpretation and belief about the situation; your mind creates the feeling, and you or your sub-personalities give it a definition. You choose to either accept and let go of the situation, or to go into emotional trauma. How deep and intense is your choice? Granted as children, we are unable to understand the consequences of how our parents treated us. But what about the children that seem to overcome almost insurmountable odds and successfully make it out of abusive families without the scars of emotional trauma? It all has to do with our viewpoint and how we respond.

An electrical current flows unimpeded through a thick copper wire, but if we run the same current through a fine wire, the wire will glow hot and may burn out. This is because the fine wire has greater resistance to the current—its ability to conduct electricity is less than the thick wire. Similarly, physical or emotional pain stems from energy meeting resistance in a meridian that is somehow blocked.

Suppose you fall down and hurt yourself. The pain you feel is real, and most people would claim that the pain cannot be released immediately. However, it is evident that pain reactions are mind-induced. Many people undergo major surgery with no anesthesia other than acupuncture. Others use hypnosis, which through autosuggestion, suppresses pain during surgery. Countless other examples demonstrate the awesome power of the mind when used properly.

Aging, too, is a state of mind, a belief that we buy into hook, line and sinker. Society and the health care and insurance industries tell us that we have increased our longevity to 75 years. That's great, but what about people in rural Tibet who live to be 125 or older? What's their secret? They are isolated from Western culture and medicine. They have no stress. Family units are close. The nuclear family is intact and there is no fight for equality that causes competition. Everyone is accepted as equal. They are vegetarians for the most part. Their water has a high mineral content. Even those over 100 get plenty of exercise. They have no air pollution. And they are not bombarded by insurance company mortality statistics.

Our body gives us wake up calls all the time, but are we awake to the message? The first time it may just be a whisper to get you to notice, then maybe a bump with pain attached. If that doesn't, it may arrange a car wreck to get your attention. Your body will get more aggressive and abrasive with each situation, and eventually, sustained denial and avoidance will result in illness, disease, or some other form of body or mind dysfunction. You can recognize the message, but first you may have to overcome denial.

If you are in denial, you may be using an addictive or dysfunctional behavior pattern to maintain control over other people in an effort to extract their conditional love and acceptance. No one has to suffer, however. Peace, happiness, harmony, joy, and unconditional love are our birthright, but most of us get love in odd and dysfunctional ways, because we were programmed about what love is during childhood. As children, if we interpret any focused attention as love, we may continue to do that as adults, and wonder why our lives do not give us what we want.

Twelve-step recovery programs often trade one addiction for another. Addiction indicates you're overdoing it and getting too much of something you don't want. Some people say they are addicted to love, but how can you become addicted to something that most people do not get enough of? Can that really be true about love? I don't think so. To me, it is relationship addiction, based on the fear of being alone.

You will follow the path and act according to the contents of your programs and their files. However, based on sheer willpower, people do successfully countermand their files and programs. But it's hard on the body/mind, however, because you create a double-bind. When your mind's program tells you, "You cannot do this particular task," but you do it anyway, it takes a lot of energy, drains your adrenal glands, and wears you out. It is much easier to clear and release the programs so that your life can flow, instead of bumping into boulders in your path.

The more stress we place on ourselves, and the more we speed up to stay with the pace of life, the more pressure we place on our mind and body. Our body/mind should function at a frequency of 12 – 18 hertz, yet most people operate between 40 – 100 hertz, which strains the adrenal glands. As the frequency increases, increased adrenaline production serves as an antidote to the "happy" brain chemicals—serotonin, interluken, interferon, etc. As a result, we can burn out and go into adrenal insufficiency, which in turn can cause Chronic Fatigue Syndrome, Epstein-Barr Syndrome, and Chronic Depression. (See Appendix for description of Body/Mind Harmonizer that will bring down the frequency and cause accelerated healing of the body.)

Chapter 8

Sub-personalities: Their Origin and Effect

I have been aware of sub-personalities for more than 15 years. Transactional Analysis talks about the five basic sub-personalities: Inner Child, Critical Parent, Survivor Self, Inner Adult, and Inner Self. These sub-personalities can have a major effect on your life, and if you operate on auto-pilot or give your power away to any of them, they will function as you and for you, projecting their agendas on your actions.

For many years, I assumed that Ego was the enemy that sabotaged our life, but when I learned about the myriad sub-personality selves and their agenda, I changed my views. We have to make friends with Ego and erase the operating systems from which the controlling sub-personalities derive their power. This is one of the most important finds we made in developing Neuro/Cellular Repatterning.

When we discovered that we were not limited to the basic five sub-personalities, we found that the personality self is composed of more than one hundred sub-personalities, each acting out a specific behavior trait. As we dug deeper into this concept, we discovered that this is what people have accepted as Ego. As we expanded our knowledge of the concept, it became a reality as we were able to change a person's personality traits, which changed his or her life path. People who were considered to have self-centered egotistic behavior could become more compassionate and supportive. Those who were nonassertive could move to a more assertive position and reclaim their personal power. Over time, we were able to show people how to reconstruct their personality so they would be more effective in their life. This is the goal of psychology but it does not work very well. It did not work for me, which was why I gave it up and began to search for a new approach.

Voice Dialogue, developed by Hal Stone, Ph.D., introduced us to disowned selves. This process uses three chairs, two for the positive and negative aspects of self, and a third in the center for the inner self, the balanced self who will generally tell the truth. But having discovered how the mind is controlled by sub-personalities and possessive beings, I now wonder exactly who we were talking to. I discovered who we were talking to as we unfolded the sub-personality pattern. Hal Stone described many of them as "disowned selves," which we had to make peace with. My feeling was that I wanted to erase these disowned selves and delete them from the files. But I found that we had to get in contact with the programs that were running them and clear them. As we were able to rewrite the scripts that we live by, we found that we could change the person's direction in life simply by installing new programs that eliminated the dysfunctional program which then would change a person's basic behavior pattern.

The five basic sub-personalities are indigenous to our mind, and everyone has these installed in the mind at birth. In the past, they were believed to be located in the Subconscious Mind. It was thought that the five were driven by Ego, which spawned the term "egotistic." However, this is erroneous because Ego has no driving force that would cause it to act egotistically. This personality trait is driven by the controller, justifier, confronter, manipulator, authority and judger sub-personalities

They are located in the Middle Self and they function autonomously, almost as a separate mind. They do, however, display what

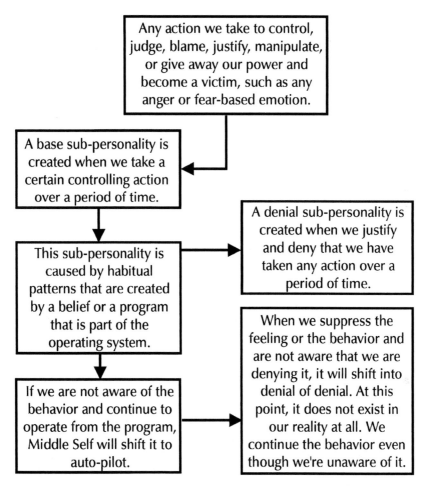

Figure 8: Creation of a sub-personality

most people mean by the term "egotistic behavior." In fact, when people are on auto-pilot, the sub-personalities run the body/mind on their own, having no real connection with Ego at all. The more we evaluated Ego, we more we found it to be simply a database for the computer, serving Subconscious Mind as librarian, secretary, and file clerk.

When we stopped confronting Ego as an adversary, it became friendly and helpful. We also discovered an interesting phenomenon: people's memories started getting better, proving that Ego was the file clerk for our memory. As we delved into this vast unknown area of the mind, we found that the makeup of the mind was as orderly and smooth-running as a well-programmed computer.

Middle Self was the area of the mind in which sub-personalities operated; at least, that was our impression until we ran into auto-pilot which has sub-personalities that we create when we let auto-pilot run our life and refuse to take responsibility. Although residing in Middle Mind, auto-pilot operates from the Conscious Mind, and we found lots of them, each driving a particular emotion. We also found that sub-personalities can drive beliefs, interpretations, feelings and programs.

People often blame the Inner Child for unruly behavior, and then deny that they have control over it. We then have to get Inner Child to grow up and stop acting like a victim. The degree to which it will fight for control depends on how much power was given to it. Survivor Self sees its role as protecting you, so it will sabotage you if it feels you are going the wrong direction. Critical Parent berates you for not doing an effective job, so that you reject yourself. This self is the most active in children because they feel they do not match up (due to parental expectations) and it spares no effort in validating any perceived shortcomings.

As we grow up, we create the judger, controller, justifier, manipulator, competitor, avoider and a myriad of anger and fear selves that run our life. And each time you run into a problem you cannot handle, your mind may create another sub-personality to deal with it. If we encounter a habit pattern that we don't want to deal with and delude ourselves, our denial creates a denial sub-personality to justify the behavior and cover it up, so that we don't even understand what we are running away from. If we try to suppress the pattern totally, the sub-personality will create a "denial of denial" sub-personality to bury it completely. We will not even recognize the behavior pattern, yet it is clearly visible to other people.

This cascade effect was one of the most significant causes of separation from self. When separation from self begins to take hold, an inner shadow sub-personality will block the person from understanding this phenomena. The more we go into denial of separation from self, more inner shadow sub-personalities are created. I have removed up to 35 inner shadow sub-personalities that were feeding negative self-talk to a client.

Sub-personalities can be up to three deep on any one subject. Not only that, dysfunctional programs and patterns often have a backup sub-personality. If these are not addressed, they will create a new program or belief driving them. We used to believe that we simply had to get to the core issue and the base cause. Now we realize that we must check for sub-personalities, too. That was not all; they have denial sub-personalities, with a back-up for each.

The hardest sub-personalities to locate are "denial of denial." Unless you're willing to face the truth and go for it, dropping all of the illusions of what you think a situation is, you cannot get to the denial sub-personalities. They are there for the very purpose of denial, so you will be blocked, making it very hard to locate them.

If you feel that you have handled a situation when, in fact, all you did was suppress the emotion, you have created denial and the issue no longer exists in your conscious mind. As it is suppressed, it will create denial of denial, and becomes lost in your mind.

We all want to live in peace, happiness, harmony and joy, with an abundance of prosperity and unconditional love, but how many really achieve that? My experience is that less than 20 percent are satisfied with their life. Many people will delude themselves into feeling they are happy when in fact, on checking with their Inner Minds, we find different answers. Furthermore, less than 25 percent of people love themselves or will allow others to love them.

How many people in serious pain are told they have to live with it or take drugs to kill the symptoms? Almost all of them, even though this statement is not true, but most doctors do not know any different. They practice what they are taught without questioning the result. The drug companies push drugs and the doctors buy the line. A few have seen the truth but not many. In truth, the medical profession is doing the best it can with the tools and knowledge available. Being open to new knowledge is blocked by control sub-personalities.

Our research into the causes of depression revealed that it is usually controlled by a sub-personality. The base cause is normally separation from self, not wanting to take responsibility, or running away from some situation you do not want to face. To avoid responsibility, your body goes into depression, which is caused by worry, anxiety, self-pity, grief, confusion, indecision or hopelessness.

The end result is that your body frequency increases and the adrenal glands release extra adrenaline. Adrenaline focuses us on "fight or flight." Once the body's need for the excess adrenaline is over, the mind signals with a shot of nor-adrenaline, the antidote and neutralizer to the adrenaline. If the adrenal glands continually kick in large amount of adrenaline to keep you functioning, you can go into adrenal insufficiency as your body frequency goes up and the brain chemicals stop production. However, adrenaline suppresses the "happy-making" brain chemicals.

Your energy is now coming from adrenaline rather than the normal sources. As this continues, the adrenal glands are overworked and slow down production. If they get down to 35 percent of normal function, the body further slows down until it goes into clinical depression and Chronic Fatigue Syndrome. Usually a person is in denial when they are in depression, so a denial sub-personality runs the auto-pilot. It then becomes very difficult to reprogram any dysfunctional patterns

At this point, you feel as though you're dying because you're operating at 30 percent or less of capacity. As every function in your body slows down, you cannot digest food properly, so you do not get the proper nutrition. Doctors cannot always diagnose what is happening, so they put it down as depression and prescribe a mind-altering drug. This gives your body a boost and allows the adrenal glands to rest, but they cannot recover because the drugs are supporting and suppressing the symptom.

The ideal body frequency is 12 – 18 hertz. In this range, the body functions at its best and will heal quickly. We have also found that rewriting programs and clearing sub-personalities is easier when the Body/Mind functions at its optimum levels. (The Body/Mind Harmonizer is an electronic device that promotes optimum functioning. See Appendix B for details.)

The first task is to locate the dysfunctional sub-personality and find out what's driving it. If it's a program, we have to find the base cause and where it's located on the body. Then we must find out to which person or to what situation the client reacted that caused the core issue. When we clear and release them, we can rewrite the operating instructions and clear the sub-personality. If it is a belief and not a reality, we can rewrite the operating instructions with a simple affirmation that clears both belief and concept.

We have found that most people have little control over their lives. I used to believe that auto-pilot was not an effective part of one's minds, so I would erase the operating system. At the time, I did not realize how little control people had over their life, so when I did so, my clients would often pass out because I had crashed their Middle Self's operating system.

If we have released all of the body-based programs, the beliefs, the core issues, and the base cause, we wondered why a program we have released often resurfaces. With discovery of the denial and denial of denial sub-personalities, we found that they could rebuild a habit pattern and the programs to run it. If any part of the file is not erased, it can be recreated and reactivated. The result is that even though we've cleared all beliefs and the programs, the denial sub-personalities can restructure and activate an old program.

Recently we discovered another file that explained why some programs get reinstalled. When we are frustrated, we find the answer quite often if we will just become quiet and listen to the direction intuitively. I did this while I was sitting in a steam room at my health club (I do much meditating in the steam room or sauna). What came to me was to look into future time-lines. Many programs can be locked into future time-lines with specific dates when they are to activate or reactivate. This was a major find as we have been able to find and clear sub-personalities that we not only put in denial-of-denial with programs, but also put in future time-lines for us to deal with in the future.

Now that we have the total picture, we've been able to totally clear a program without reoccurrence. For a complete list of the sub-personalities and a description of the release process, see Chapter 15.

Chapter 9

Meta-Communication

Meta-Communication is the ultimate form of body language. Our body projects our thoughts and feelings all around us without our knowledge. Your body is talking, but are you listening?

Did you know that who you are precedes you everywhere you go? You project out to everyone you meet exactly how you feel about yourself. If others are observant, they will be able to form an impression of how you feel about yourself before you say a word. You may think you can put on a front and fool people about who you are, but your mind always betrays you when you try to put on a cover. It always tells the truth even if you live in an illusion or delude yourself into thinking you can hide or block other people from seeing who you are or how you feel. An intuitive person can observe exactly how you feel about yourself.

Your mind projects the basic interpretation of your self-worth and your self-confidence to those intuitive enough to pick it up. This is one of the most important features of your mind that must be mastered, and the only way to do it is to release all the feelings that defeat you. To do this, you have to work through the childhood feelings that cause you to feel you are not all right. This is described elsewhere in this book, so suffice to say that one of the major programs that blocks us from achieving any end is, "I am not entitled to ...."

This block applies to anything that we want in life, and the mere act of wanting something guarantees that you will not get it. You will deny yourself money, fame, success, acceptance, functional relationships, the ideal position or job and many other things, because you feel you are not entitled to whatever it may be. *You cannot want and have at the same time.*

Suppose you apply for a loan to buy a house, a car, or any large value item and are turned down. You cannot see why: I dressed the proper way, and I did all the right things, yet I was turned down. A friend goes in to get the same loan. He or she is not dressed in "banker's clothes," they don't have your income or your credit rating, yet they get the loan. Why, you ask?

It actually has nothing to do with how you presented yourself externally. You are presenting yourself to a person who has to feel comfortable with your trustworthiness. The meta-communication that you transmit influences the loan officer's decision more than any other "credentials" you can present. It's not how you look that matters, but how you present yourself on an inner level that counts. You may complain, "That's unfair; how can this happen?"

It's all about recovery of your self-worth, and letting go of fear, control and manipulation. It's about being willing and able to forgive everyone in your life, about not harboring blame or resentment, about not projecting "victim" in your meta-communication.

The person who exudes self-confidence, self-worth and self-esteem is interpreted by other people as a more trustworthy person. Generally they are more ethical and will follow through with the responsibilities they have taken on. The person who lacks these qualities will generally project an "I'm not all right; I'm not entitled to …" attitude that is clearly evident to people who have to evaluate other people for a living.

Quite often a person with low self-esteem will make poor decisions in how they handle their life. Twenty years ago, if I had to purchase something, due to my earlier programming I would unerringly choose a vendor who would take advantage of me, or a product that was guaranteed to fail. It was as though I was signaling, "I'm a sucker who will let you take advantage of me." It must have been written all over me. Unfortunately, we attract other people to validate how we feel about ourselves and teach us a lesson. I got angry at myself when I discovered what I was doing, but I kept on doing it until I finally woke up to the fact that I was creating it all.

When we take our personal power back, begin to operate from high self-esteem, and validate ourselves, people will no longer take advantage of us. If we set ourselves up as doormats, people will obligingly walk all over us. When I recovered my self-worth, confidence and self-esteem, I stopped projecting this negative image. Suddenly, people changed their attitude about me, yet they did not know they had done so. People started helping me instead of ripping me off. I had become a different person, and walked into another life.

We unknowingly project our self-image to whomever will listen. What you say or do makes no difference unless you work on your innermost feelings about who you are at a deep level. Most people have denial sub-personalities covering and suppressing who they really are, so they have no way of uncovering the cause. Getting in contact with the programs that are defeating us takes committed, disciplined work. Most people run on autopilot, unwilling to spend time or money to get to the cause and clear it.

Most of my clients who claim to be working on spiritual growth have no idea what their meta-communication is projecting out to other people, regardless of what they say about themselves.

New York University's Department of Psychology conducted one of the most definitive studies on meta-communication. In conjunction with the New York Police Department, 50 men and women convicted of robbery, molestation, rape, attack and many other crimes were asked to study people picked at random—many of whom had already been victims of some sort—and select those they would most likely choose as victims. Not surprisingly, only the former victims were chosen, those who had been attacked in the past. Furthermore, the "victims" selected most frequently had been attacked many times before. The psychological profiles of the victims and non-victims revealed great differences in self-worth and good feelings about themselves.

Prior to 1981, if I got stuck with a defective product, I would say, "That is a lesson and I should let go and release it." But after I had a new interpretation, the next time I had to take a product back and get credit for it—a defective screen door—I accepted the responsibility to reclaim my power. I had a new attitude, too. My intent was not a credit or refund, but to make a point. When the clerk realized that I was neither blaming nor being a victim, she quickly gave me a credit. I didn't attack her or the company, even though she volunteered that they'd had many doors returned. The important thing was that I was not complaining or attacking; I had no need to control or manipulate. She recognized that because I wasn't playing the victim and yelling at her, she didn't have to protect herself and could allow herself the vulnerability to admit this was a defective product that they no longer carried. My meta-communication allowed her to respond positively to my request and the outcome was mutually beneficial.

When you take responsibility for your actions and stand up for yourself, people will take notice and help you. This has happened many times, even when someone refuses to repair or accept a product back. Admittedly, it doesn't always work, and I have had to resort to small claims court a few times.

Our "denial" sub-personalities often set us up and steer us away from the very situations that would help us. Our "justifier" sub-personality will convince us that we did the right thing. We will follow its path not knowing that we lost our way, until we reach the point of pain (physical or emotional).

Even though we have not broken through their barriers of denial, clients will offer excuses to justify why they are not seeing me anymore. I clearly see the meta-communication, yet I cannot break through their denial for them, unless they decide that they want to. Many clients truly desire to break through, but their minds have been so programmed to operate in a certain way that they have to really discipline themselves to watch every thought and statement.

The only way out is to get into recovery, take responsibility, and let go of all blame, control and manipulation. Control is the biggest addiction there is, and most of us use it covertly and overtly. Being able to blame someone else for taking advantage of you creates a comfortable sense of security.

Chapter 10

There Is a Way Out: Healing Miracles

There is a way out. Recovery is possible. Dysfunctional behavior, illness and disease are a state of mind. Let me reiterate that this process is not spiritual healing. We are following rules that produce the same results every time if people will commit themselves and discipline themselves to follow the directions.

Whatever you believe forms your reality, and generates the programs and patterns that drive your life. You may not even believe that you created your life as it is, but are you willing to unload all your false beliefs and transform your life now? *There is no other time than now.* If you think you will do it when you are ready, you may wait until your next life. You have to make the decision and there is no better time than now. Do it now and see what happens; you have nothing to lose except your discomfort. You can get on with your mission in life.

Of course, change causes fear because most people would rather suffer than change. If you are in denial, you may not even be aware that you are not on the path. Sometimes playing victim can get you many rewards—you can control other people and manipulate them to get attention even though you say you don't want to. *You can be in denial of denial which gives you the illusion that you are living your truth—"I am all right the way I am"—and nobody can break that illusion except you.* You must first recognize the illusion.

How do you confront your illusions? There is a way out if you want to reclaim your personal power and take responsibility. Nobody can heal you; it's all on your shoulders. When you decide that life is not working the way you are now, all you have to do is decide to confront the delusion, the umbrella you're living under. Very seldom can people see their own illusions because denial obscures them. Some people have been able to break through the denial themselves, but it takes tremendous personal power to reclaim responsibility and be willing to fly into new territory. It is like jumping off a cliff and knowing you can fly. I describe this as the "Jonathan Livingston Seagull lesson," because you're jumping into the unknown.

Transformation requires you to jump out of the nest and fly. Looked at from the outside, it may seem simple, but trying to fly while holding onto the fear of letting go will bring up fear of the unknown. You can find many reasons not to fly, such as blaming other people for causing your reluctance. In an effort to stop you from threatening your security, your mind will set up myriad reasons why this is happening. *Remember, your mind considers security the status quo.* Anything that threatens the security must be prevented.

If you have been on auto-pilot for most of your life, reclaiming your personal power is a threat to the power structure in your mind. However, when you deprogram all the denial sub-personalities, the results may seem miraculous, because there is no resistance to change. Most people, though, need help in confronting the programs that are controlling their life. Some people will seek help in the form of psychotherapy or some other form of counseling. But very few practitioners can get to the base cause and core issues because they're not trained to go beyond the surface issues presented by the client.

I have found that about 15 percent of the population love themselves and can receive love from others. So how do we overcome these tragic odds? By rewriting the program, by locating the base cause, the core issue and with whom you participated in the situation to put you on your current path. To release the program/

belief, we have to locate how you reacted in the base cause/core issue situation. How you are currently handling it in your life will show us how we have to release the program. We then form an affirmation to describe the situation, and move into loving and forgiving those involved, and loving and forgiving yourself for allowing the situation to happen. Bingo, the condition is healed and released. If this seems simple, in fact, it is. All we do is guide you to reprogram your mind so it can create a different response. To many people in their condition, however, this seems impossible.

Miracles do happen every day. Transformation is instantaneous, recovery from anything is possible. I experience at least twelve to fifteen miracles a year. Why not make yours one. All it takes is your desire, commitment and willingness to consistently discipline yourself to follow through with a plan to take responsibility. Pain will disappear instantly when you recognize your "alrightness."

You have your life back! Self-esteem, self-confidence, and self-worth return. You never lost it; you just wrote over it with dysfunctional programming. When we erase and rewrite the programs, the real you emerges. You came here to be a spiritual being taking on a physical body to learn some lessons and let go of karma. Why not get on with it? There is no better time than *now!* But if you wait until you feel ready, your denial may cause it to be delayed and it may not happen in this lifetime. You can make the commitment now. No one is stopping you except you. This is the right time. There will never be a better time than right now. The only limitations are your own beliefs and denials that create the limitations. Yes, it will take some hard work and a strong commitment, but yes, it can be done. You can be a miracle, you have the ability. All you have to do is let go of anger, control, manipulation, authority over, judgment, justification, righteousness, rebellion, the need to please people for acceptance, and the addiction to these types of behavioral patterns.

The most complex thing for people to understand is that we never lose anything positive or negative. The sub-personalities and the programs just go into denial or get written over. A program or habit pattern is not deleted by writing over it, as with computer files. When you erase, and overwrite programs such as indigenous operational programs, they can immediately reconfigure and remain operational unless you clear the belief and sub-personality, too. We discovered this when we became aware that the belief, program or pattern reactivated and became operational again. You must lock up negative programs and sub-personalities in the history archives of your mind. By doing this, we have secured the program forever. It can not reconfigure or reactivate.

Chapter 14 presents case studies that show how all this takes place.

Chapter 11

Neuro/Cellular Repatterning: The Practice of Psychoneuroimmunology

Disclaimer

We are not practicing any form of medical practice nor do we diagnose or prescribe any medicines of any kind. We simply ask the body/mind to reveal to us the base causes and core issues. When we find the defective programming, we erase defective beliefs, programs and habit patterns. Then we then restructure the mind's programs that control illness, diseases and behavioral dysfunction.

Neuro/Cellular Repatterning (N/CR) is a holographic body-based spiritual psychotherapy process that uses neuro-kinesiology and affirmations with love and forgiveness as the basic modality. Love and forgiveness are the only two modalities that will cause healing to happen.

N/CR will be one of the healing processes in the new millennium, because it holds the promise of healing any dysfunction, illness, disease or emotional/mental problems without pain, drugs or surgery. No diagnosis is needed, just recognition of the base cause and core issue. When you locate and release the base cause and core issue driving the dysfunction, healing begins to happen automatically.

Any side-issues that have contributed to the dysfunction will also come up during a session. They, too, will have to be released. Programs, beliefs and interpretations that drive sub-personalities must be addressed, too. The body does not lie; it always tells the truth if you are clear and not in denial. If denial exists, we may have to deprogram the denial to get a specific answer. Denial of denial can block any recognition of a program. A sub-personality is usually driving the denial. If that case, we have to work through the fear that caused a person to suppress the information. We have to be open to anything that may come up.

The basic concept in N/CR is to release the causes and core issues blocking the client from the truth. When we see who we really are and recognize that no matter what happened in the past, we are all right as we are, we can reclaim our personal power and empower ourselves to take responsibility for our lives. We can then begin to love and forgive ourselves. This work is not about doing lip service to make it look acceptable. It is about telling the truth about ourselves and accepting others as they are without the need for control, authority or manipulation over anybody.

When we understand the awesome power of the Conscious Rational Mind, Middle Self and the Subconscious Mind to disable our immune system and body's functioning, we will see how disease is created. In an analogy to computers, the Subconscious Mind is a central computer that networks with each of the personal cellular computers that perform the tasks programmed into them by their DNA. Any false beliefs, concepts, attitudes and interpretations in the system will create programs that cause cells to create life or death. The response is automatic, without conscious thought, and if we are not control as the programmer, then the program is installed without our consent or even awareness.

Your body is your mind, and in computer language, it is also the hardware. The 'software' is any program installed in the mind. The Instinctual Mind is just that: if you go into survival mode, it takes over. It has no ability to think or make rational decisions or place sensory input in the "database." The only program it has is to keep us alive or cause death if an "I want to die program" gets installed.

The Conscious Mind is the programmer. However, it, too, can hold false beliefs and concepts you are not aware of. If you do not question these beliefs, they will run your life. *YOU, the programmer* of the conscious mind, must be on track all the time. If you 'walk out' and go on auto-pilot, the Middle Self's sub-personalities, along with auto-pilot, will take over and run your life because somebody must always be at the helm.

We are finding that people are separating from their body in increasing numbers each year, a phenomenon we call "graying out," in which you are intermittently out of your body, which causes dexterity problems, fogged vision, etc. "Browning out" can cause memory lapse but you can still function. "Blacking out" happens when a person loses consciousness momentarily—something I feel is the cause of many single-car wrecks—because it has happened to me twice.

In our practice, a 12-month test found that most people are running on auto-pilot more than 85 percent of the time. Our intention is to empower people to take 100 percent control of their lives. We succeed most of the time.

Hundreds of clients have experienced seeming miracles with N/CR, including amazing spontaneous releases of disease, emotional dysfunction and genetic defects. Yet, others didn't respond well, or the dysfunction would return. Why that happened mystified me for many years. Recently, we discovered that if a denial or denial-of-denial program or sub-personality exists, it will not be detected unless we ask for that specific program. When we clear the base cause and the core issues without checking for denial programs, they can replicate the exact same illness, disease or behavioral conditions.

At that point, I realized I was not 'doing" it, that we were not "healers" or "therapists." We are here only to teach people how to love themselves, receive love and empower themselves to take control of their lives. If you can take responsibility and make that shift in consciousness, permanent healing will follow. A therapist cannot change the holographic image a client holds about self, but only help the client make the spiritual/mental shift, thereby causing the healing. If the client does not make that shift, the healing process will give them only a temporary release. All we can do is help our clients recognize the cause or core issues and release the emotional charge. We can help them to preprogram the situation and rewrite new scripts, accepting the past, and loving and forgiving themselves and others. As facilitators, we cannot install the programs, but we can help by developing the script and using affirmations to install it. Acceptance is up to the client. It works 98 percent of time, but there will always be clients who resist.

N/CR will work in spite of itself, because we are not working with the Conscious Mind. As a result, we are able to duplicate the process in 95 percent of cases. All programs seem to be the same in all people; there may be different responses, but they all have the same result.

Many times, the Instinctual Mind will try to keep you in survival mode, as it is originally programmed to do. In an N/CR session, we ask it to abide by our will and work with us. Since you are the scriptwriter, producer and director of all the shows in your life, we ask it to let you come out of the wings and take center stage. When you are the lead in your play, the Subconscious Mind will cooperate with you; this is accomplished by talking to the Instinctual Mind with an affirmation.

The Middle Self is another matter altogether. If the Middle Self or a sub-personality interferes, we use a different approach to make friends with your Middle Self, so that it won't sabotage you. N/CR accesses the Middle Self programming and gets it to recognize you as the computer programmer and director. If it does not want to step aside, we can erase the operating system and replace it with a new one that is not contaminated with controlling beliefs and concepts. Quite often we have to also erase sub-personalities that are controlling and operating in Middle Self.

I have found that it is not the modality that causes healing to happen, since many allopathic and alternative therapies have claimed provable, visible healing. However, they cannot explain why remission happens or how to duplicate the process with any regularity. There is no such thing as a cure by removing the physical result. True healing happens when the program that causes the dysfunction is cleared, along with all the beliefs, concepts, attitudes and interpretations that drive the sub-personality is erased that initially created the cellular or mental malfunction.

The effectiveness of a practitioner depends upon his/her ability to get in touch with clients' "feeling self." You must set up trust, so the client feels that you care and love them; this is what allows healing to take place. Healing is governed by only one law: LOVE, and it works every time. My study with *A Course In Miracles* formed part of the base, as well as *The Healing Touch*, by Dolores Kruegar.

Psychiatrists, doctors, psychologists and practitioners recognize the need to release negative emotions, yet few of them know how to do this. The methods they are taught are not effective; the training I went through was woefully inadequate. N/CR is a controlled process which will get to the core issue. Double blind treatments with different practitioners working with N/CR have shown that each practitioner has virtually the same experiences. All fear appears on the left side of the body; all anger appears on the right. Rejection deposits along the spine; we have uncovered over sixty individual basic locations for specific emotional, dysfunctional programs (see charts in Chapter 3).

As if the Universe is trying to give us the answer, many doctors and medical researchers are discovering the answers to the puzzle of healing. In a *Discovery* magazine article, "A Bug in the System," scientists reported discovering the causes of a disease syndrome. They labeled it a "genetic defect," but offered no cure, prognosis or correction; People lose their eyesight, yet they cannot locate the cause except that "It must be genetic." The cellular breakdown is caused by the cell's mitochondria losing its ability to process and absorb nutrients. The cellular structure begins to break down from inability to assimilate nutrients and begins to malfunction. Their interpretation is that the cells are dying because of a genetic defect.

Whatever diagnosis the researchers come up with becomes the disease. This explains why healing works with N/CR; it erases the cellular memory of the rejection, lack of love, etc., and helps the cell recover its original blueprint, so it begins to rebuild a new healthy cell. In effect, we are reprogramming DNA in the cellular computer software. This is the key to healing.

Many people recognize this and are developing programs and processes to perform a DNA shift. I have my doubts that these processes work since they are not getting to the basic program that exists in the cellular memory. The DNA is the software of each cell. *You can't use general affirmations to rewrite the software. I have found they must be specific to the individual issue and must contain very specific language and wording in an exact format to reprogram the DNA.*

With counseling, physical therapy and almost all alternative therapies, you can remove the energy causing the pain or discomfort. But, if you do not go further to locate the root cause, it will be a simple, symptomatic release. We have simply masked the problem until the same catalyst or stimulus reappears and the emotional energy builds up again, reactivating the disease, illness or dysfunctional emotional program.

With N/CR, we locate the base cause, core issue, uncovering the belief and/or the Subconscious Mind's program. When an experience is filed, it creates a record and program, with energy that makes small chemical changes in the body. Each program records how we reacted and handled the incident the first time. Each time we encounter this program, we build more patterns with instructions on how we will handle future situations. If it is a strong habit pattern, a sub-personality will be created to drive the program and belief. Eventually these chemical changes will cause a physical breakdown in the body. To release the dysfunctional emotion and the program, we have to understand the cause, and the reason you reacted in the manner you did. When we understand the dialogue between Conscious and Subconscious Minds, the Middle Self and your body, we can disconnect that conversation and release it. Then we erase the program's operating instructions, destroy the patterns and file the record, pattern and program in the Subconscious Mind's history archives. At this point, the emotional energy is released and the behavior program is no longer accessible to you.

At the physical level, the cellular memory is released, which allows the muscle to return to its original form. The short-circuit in the meridian that caused the muscle to go into contraction from emotional trauma is released. At the same time, the neuro-pathway patterns created from the experience are released and erased. The original program surfaces in the Subconscious Mind which allows the electrical transmissions to the muscles to be reestablished in their original format, and the pain is gone.

In the case of a life-threatening, dysfunctional program, the endocrine system's original programs are restored, so the immune system can rebuild the T-cells, and the leukocyte count increases to destroy the dysfunctional invading cells. All the physical programs are controlled by your mind's central computer, the Subconscious Mind.

Illness or disease is often caused by programming from some authority figure who told you that you are subject to a hereditary disease syndrome. If you do not cancel such a statement, your mind will accept that statement as a belief. This belief will cause the described effect, disease, illness or dysfunction to materialize and become a reality now or at some future date or age. Your mind responds to the program's input to the data base and will cause the information to be written into the record. These beliefs can be released by a simple affirmation, but again, it must be specific to the individual belief. We also must release the person who caused it, loving and forgiving them, too. In all cases, the belief/program/pattern must be locked up in the archives so it cannot reactivate or be accessed in the future.

Beliefs cause major illusions. To clear beliefs, we have to test for denial and denial-of-denial. Programs are often disguised by denials (see *Chapter 5: Beliefs, and Cause and Effect*).

Most denials are driven by a sub-personality that covers the belief or program. When we get these out of the way, we can go for the base cause and the core issue.

Quite often a person will create their own illness, disease, dysfunction or even death to slow themselves down or to escape a particular situation. These are the most difficult situations to work with in N/CR because they always involve denial, and in some cases denial-of-denial. To get to the core issue, first we have to release the denial. I have no problem in getting to the cause as I can see the issue very clearly. The challenge is to get the client to let go of the denial. We plant a seed in the mind by going through the affirmations for denial, but if that seed does not sprout and open up the awareness to cause, we get nowhere. The client has to be able to recognize the issue before we can do any releasing. If the client continues to deny the cause, the situation will persist.

Often, frequent sessions will break the barrier, but some clients will deny that they're resisting because they have walked out to the point that auto-pilot sub-personalities are running their life. This is especially common with alcohol addiction. Alcoholics have to come to clarity with themselves before they can admit that alcohol is a poison to their system and they are an alcoholic. It is similar to Multiple Personality Disorder (a.k.a. Dissociative Identity Disorder) since the Conscious Rational Mind is non-functional. The controlling sub-personality is in total control and may block any release. We can usually get around the blockage by working with the Middle Self.

The body is a hologram, and we must address all levels at the same time. We must work with physical, mental, emotional, and spiritual levels simultaneously; otherwise the treatment will be symptomatic and temporary. N/CR will access the root cause, because it requires the practitioner to get in contact with the "feeling self." By doing so, she/he can listen to information in the client's Subconscious Mind, which the mind has deposited in muscles/acupuncture points. The practitioner uses acupuncture points as switches to turn on the video/ audio and allow the mind to bring the picture and experience to the front. (This is where the similarity with other therapies stops.)

Since the practitioner listens to body/mind, and goes directly to base cause, we get clear insights as to the cause of the dysfunction. By describing the situation which caused the dysfunction, then using an affirmation and asking the client to repeat it, the blockage is released. My experience with Science of Mind helped me understand the importance of the power of affirmation in releasing and filing the record, program and pattern.

Despite what many people want to believe, we are all clairvoyant. It is not a gift, nor are only some blessed with this gift. We all have it, we just have to reclaim it. We all were capable as children, but were told such things as "You're seeing things that do not exist," or "This is the work of the devil." Needless to say, we lost the ability due to non-use. Our educational system denied this ability so it was lost. What would happen if children were intuitive and the teachers were not? Teachers could not control the children because the latter would know the truth without having to pay attention. I was frequently sent to the nurse's office because I was sleeping in the class, yet I would ace the test even though I'd missed the class—frustrating for the teacher.

Regardless of technique, most therapy today focuses on releasing or suppressing symptoms; unfortunately that will not heal the body. Most practitioners expect some form of remission, cure or healing, but if you do not access the root cause, any outcome will be temporary and symptomatic. The body will always tell the truth, no matter what we believe or even if we choose not to believe it. We always find that fear, anger and rejection are the base causes, yet, as clients, we are always trying to blame some outside incident, person, or virus. The mind can create any disease it chooses, but the only thing that heals is love. With N/CR, the client is allowed a safe space to learn how to love self and release the blockages in the body. The self is therefore freed to receive the basic needs of all people: love, acceptance, approval and a feeling of being all right. These lead to self-esteem and self-worth.

Many people recognize the need to release emotional/physical cellular memory, but very few achieve results. Cathartic release does not always indicate that the base cause or core issue has been revealed. Disease and dysfunctional emotional behavior patterns are directly caused by the inability to accept oneself as all right and the refusal to give and receive love! Love can heal anything. To reverse the disease process, we must understand unconditional love and accept it.

When I discovered N/CR, it was difficult to define. I realized that everything hinged on what the mind accepts as truth. I gave up on psychology because how could the therapist describe a situation to me if all he has to go on is his limited experience which could be blocked by denial and illusion on his part. I searched for a process that could get to the base cause of dysfunction without having to spend hours trying to dig out the cause from a client who couldn't even understand it in the first place. Most people don't know what their mind has stored, let alone understand it. But I still did not connect my physical pain as emotional dysfunction within the programs in my mind. I thought all physical problems had only physical origins; at least that's what doctors told me. Yet they did not understand why my spine was deteriorating; their prognosis was that I would end in a wheelchair. The lack of specific cause baffled them; they saw my body deteriorating but no physical cause.

To me, psychology seemed to fix blame on someone or something unknown. This was in the late 1970s and I didn't believe we had to be victims of another person's reaction. At the time, I didn't know that my body was continually dialoging with me, but if I'd listened, it would have revealed the causes. So I turned to alternative healing and studied Chinese and Tibetan Medicine, and that helped a little. Homeopathy was too slow.

All told, I studied over 20 alternative forms of therapy; some released a little of the pain, but it was not permanent. In my training with Paul Solomon, we approached psychology from a holistic, spiritual aspect—a totally different slant from my original training. It answered some of my questions and helped me understand the dialogue, but it didn't heal my body. In a workshop, Ronald Beesley showed me how the body stores the memory and the basics of re-moving it. I now had the tools to integrate spiritual psychology with body/mind therapy. This became the link, which I incorporated as the basis of N/CR and my counseling.

Physical dysfunction reveals *itself* but not its *causes*. Emotional and mental pain is non-tangible, which makes it difficult to locate and work with. I was not aware that my belief system had sup-pressed emotional programs that were causing my physical prob-lem. Until John Bradshaw's *Dysfunctional Family* programs on TV, few people understood this problem.

I termed this process "Cellular Repatterning" because we were releasing the imbedded cellular memory from past experiences. Each cell has a memory of the perfect image of how it can regen-erate itself. If there is no dysfunctional negative overlay of emo-tional energy blocking, all cellular structures will regenerate perfectly from the blueprint, each time the cells are rebuilt. I added the "neuro" prefix in 1988 when I discovered that we were eras-ing the pattern used by the neurological system to keep muscles in trauma from past negative emotional experiences.

There is hope. Recovery is possible in every case. The only catch is the desire to take control and discipline self to do what it takes. I am a walking example of a miracle, as are many of my clients who literally shifted their belief and were healed in min-utes. Some took days; others gradually improved over a few years. It depends on a willingness to let go of attachment to the cause and the core issues that have manifested the dysfunction. *All of them are the same: the root cause in any dysfunction of the body or the mind is anger, fear or rejection, which results in lack of love.* When the connection to Source is restored or reconnected, love can be-gin to heal the body/mind.

Need for control is the most widespread addiction we have today. It is insidious in the way we react to it, both as therapists and clients. If you are not in recovery, it is not an issue; you cannot recognize the symptom as the illusion, and denial will mask it so perfectly that you simply cannot see it. Many people in recovery don't recognize it as an issue. If we have an expectation or want to control a program, a meeting, or a person's response, we need to control everyone to get attention. A person who needs validation from the outside interprets any concentrated form of attention as love. Many people will even hurt themselves in accidents or cause illness and disease to get love. It is not actually unconditional love, but any form of attention will do. We will suffer abuse both physical and emotional to get attention. However, when it is conditional, love has an elusive feeling.

As a therapist, I can only guide and help clients understand the causes and core issues that are causing the dysfunction in their lives, but if they cannot receive love, or love themselves, how do they receive it? If love does not exist in their reality, how do they recover self-esteem and self-worth, let alone heal themselves? However, just explaining the cause does not change the program or pattern; it will continue on until it is released from the body and mind together.

In the past, we assumed when we cleared the programs, patterns and records, that was all that was needed. Now we recognize that after we clear the programs, etc., we have to check the Middle Self to see if there are any residual beliefs about the situation stored deep in the Middle Self. The intricacies of how the mind stores information is truly amazing. We can now understand how easy it is for people bent on controlling to use mind control to affect people without their awareness.

There is a way out of the mire that bogs us down. We must address the old Catch-22; we must first commit to taking responsibility to take our power back. Only then, when we reconnect with Source—the presence of God within—can miracles do happen. Only then can we accept unconditional love from self and from others.

Love is the primary ingredient in healing; without love present, healing does not happen. You may get symptom relief but not true healing. That is why doctors describe a person who apparently has been cured to be "in remission." You cannot cure anything. But, when you release the program, belief and the sub-personality driving it, you will be healed totally and permanently. The situation will never return or re-manifest, because it has nothing to recreate it.

The challenge is: *"Are you ready to drop all your beliefs about what has happened in the past and be in the present moment?"* You may say that you believe in holistic alternative therapy. That may be true at the conscious mind level, but are your other minds aligned with that belief? Often there are programs and beliefs that are grounded in the medical model, and if that denial exists, so will doubt and skepticism that will block healing every time. You have to be willing to follow directions and accept what your body/mind reveals during a treatment session. Remember, you are the programmer and the computer operator. All I can do as a practitioner is to develop the software in the form of an affirmation and hand it to you. You have to install it by repeating the affirmation. If we are successful in replacing the old program with the new, miracles will happen. It is a mechanical effect. It happens every time; we successfully rewrite the old script and install a new one.

N/CR is an eclectic process gleaned from many other processes and therapies, and contains many elements that work together to create miracles every week. Are you ready for one in your life?

(See Chapter 15 for information on how to actually conduct an N/CR session.)

The Transition to Psychoneuroimmunology

About five years ago, I had heard about the concept of PNI but it did not register because it was a medical concept. Now that I have researched PNI, I discovered it was right in line with Neuro/Cellular Repatterning.

In 1974 Robert Adler, a psychiatrist and instructor at the University of Rochester Medical School, became interested in how the brain interacted with the body and the immune system. In 1977, the Dept. of Behavioral Medicine was established at Yale University to research PNI. In their research over the years, they found what I have contended since I begin working in this field—that the body/mind is an integrated unit. What affects one part will have an effect on all aspects of the body. Here we are 25 years later, and they have yet to introduce the concept of PNI into medical or psychological practice. Some practitioners claim to be using it, yet I have found from what I have read of their work that it is hit-and-miss. Which brings in the "placebo effect."

The placebo effect depends on clients' *belief* in the product or the practitioner. If they accept the effectiveness of the practitioner's work and/or the product, it will work. This will be covered in depth in my new book.

We are in the forefront of a paradigm shift in alternative medicine. In an attempt to understand immuno-regulatory function, converging data from different disciplines have provided compelling evidence. Like any other system operating in the effort to create homeostasis, the body, and the immune and endocrine systems are integrated with other psycho-physiological processes. What they found is that the brain interacts with the body. Bingo! We have a new avenue to research. But, at this point they have not found how to control the interactions in this stimulus response immuno-regulatory system.

The battle lines seem to be building as the conventional orthodox researchers have bristled at the concept that there is a connection between the brain and the immune system. Despite the replicated studies that have found such a link, the resistance is building. Critics claim they have yet to find a biological mechanism linking the two systems. Adler states that does not bother him as there are many medical and psychological phenomena where we have not been able to define the precise mechanisms. In a keynote presentation before the American Immunological Association, he said, "If we could put the concepts of PNI to work, it would have a depressive effect on the practices of the audience. But I assure you that this would not happen as people do not want to take responsibility for their health and we have not found a way to build a person's self-image to put PNI to work in an effective manner yet."

~ ~ ~

Many researchers are finding that psychology, medicine, religion and spirituality overlap. In some cases they find that people with a strong faith and belief in religion and/or spirituality seem to recover faster from illness. People who tend to be enthusiastic, happy and optimistic seem to recover faster also. In their research, they are finding that the Pavlovian studies of many years ago tend to bear out the facts that people who recognize a negative factor will avoid it. This finding tends to support recovery and preventive health, so they are going around the merry-go-round trying to find the answers, but they cannot see them yet. We may be able to make a breakthrough in getting medical science to accept our paradigm and the process of N/CR following publication of my new book, *The Body/Mind Medicine Connection: PsychoNeuro-Immunogy In Practice* that will document and describe how we approach every form of illness, disease and behavioral dysfunction. It will also document preventive practices to avoid the above, besides being a compendium of ways to create and maintain perfect health. It will cover all methods to build psychological, mental, physical and spiritual balance in one's life.

We will see if this breaks into the field of medical and psychological practices. We have the answers in Neuro/Cellular Repatterning. We can prove without a doubt that the mind does control the body functions and we can heal anything if the person is willing to reprogram the mind's functions. Not only that, we can create a balance whereby a person can avoid stress, and physical/mental breakdowns. We have built the wellness model and we can put it to work with 100 percent effectiveness.

Basically PNI is the study of the interrelationship and the link between the brain (mind) and the immune/endocrine systems. The sympathetic and the autonomic nervous systems are the major carriers, along with the brain chemicals neuropeptides and the cytokinins. These are bi-directional in their action. If you feel good and have a positive mental image of yourself, they support your endocrine and immune systems. If you are pessimistic and have negative feelings about yourself, they work against you and suppress your immune and endocrine systems.

Scientific researchers are trying to create a wellness model that will support a positive mental image and thereby create health and wellness. The only problem is that they are missing the main point. The mind runs on programs and you cannot force a pattern on a person who has negative programs breaking them down. Visualizations and biofeedback can help but will not change the programs. A few people can rewrite programs by practicing a belief repeatedly until it overwrites the dysfunctional program. That does not mean that the base cause has been cleared, so the program could be recreated at a later date. This takes time and few people will discipline themselves to spend time to follow through. Simonton's work has had a marginal success with cancer over the last 25 years. Some medical doctors, however, are beginning to experiment with PNI and a few have discovered that all healing is placebo effect. A doctor I met at Book Expo America had written a book on placebo effect. He claimed he was 50 percent more effective now since he began using sugar pills and saline water than when he practiced allopathic medicine.

Chapter 12

Biofeedback: A New Therapeutic Process

In conventional therapy, it is impossible to break through the belief systems created by illusions since most people seldom know what the base causes are. If they do have some understanding, it usually is not accurate unless they have done considerable processing. Even then they may not understand denial.

It is difficult to get a person to go back to painful feelings that are completely blocked by Middle Self or protective programs. If they can, we find they go back into the *emotion* rather than the *feeling*. Most people generally block recall of negative childhood trauma experiences; I see no need to dredge up more pain. We have to break through the belief systems that were created by protective illusions. We can then release them with love and forgiveness.

With N/CR, we are able to work with the subconscious mind to help reprogram the dysfunctional programs and behavior patterns. Occasionally with N/CR, we thought we had been blocked by the Ego or subconscious programming. The control programming was actually a Middle Self sub-personality. So we used biofeedback as a lie detector. With biofeedback, we could access any program or pattern in the body/mind without blocking or barriers. We could see a spread in the light bars when we were running into resistance. At the time we did not know what the resistance was. Now we do.

In 1991, Dr. John Craig introduced me to a new way of using biofeedback. Most people would identify biofeedback as a way to train yourself to handle stress or learn how to control the body's reactions such as heart rate. This again is symptomatic treatment, because you are controlling the result. You are the victim of the stress until you locate the core issue and release the cause. If you simply manipulate a symptom with behavior modification, it will rise again when you least expect it. Our intention is to get to the base cause and the core issues which are causing the lack of direction in life, disease, dysfunctional behavior, emotional/ physical pain, anger, fear, or mental/physical discomfort.

We use biofeedback as just another tool to access the base cause and the core issues that are causing dysfunction. However, we are using it in a totally different way, similar to a polygraph or lie detector. The difference is we don't care whether a person is telling the truth because they very seldom know the actual cause. We use a dual-channel biofeedback machine to track the Conscious and Subconscious Minds' responses to the questions we ask. During treatment, it indicates if the actual behavior pattern was released or if the Middle Self is blocking the release. Our intention is to locate irrational, illogical, self defeating, destructive and dysfunctional behavior patterns that are locked in the subconscious mind.

Biofeedback proved helpful in finally getting my Middle Self to understand that it had a contract with me, that it was fighting a losing battle, and that if it won the battle, it would kill my body and in turn destroy itself. I was able to demonstrate that it was created with the Body/Mind. Since Middle Self did not have any connection with my Soul, it could not transcend the body. So it decided that it wanted to continue to live and create a new life with me. We came to a successful conclusion with a win-win for both of us. It finally decided to stop the battle for control and power over me. We feel this process is the next step in breaking the barriers to total personal transformation. If you haven't come face-to-face with your Middle Self and its sub-personalities yet, it will happen. If your sub-personalities are running your life, you have a battle on your hands to reclaim control.

The key to healing is always stored in the Subconscious Mind. Illness is always caused by self-rejection and lack of love. Many times a person has totally blocked the trauma so well that we cannot locate the cause. The challenge is in accessing painful traumatic experiences. If a client cannot remember an incident, how do you access and process the issue? Most people will try to describe what they feel is the cause, but they tend to block out past painful traumatic experiences. Many people have been in therapy for up to 30 years with many cathartic releases but very little change in their emotional/mental behavior.

Are we actually getting to the core issue and releasing it? Doctors will tell patients, "You have to live with your pain," or "We can't do anything for you." That may be their truth based on their training, but we don't buy this at all. If you can locate the base causes and the core issues, you can heal any dysfunction of the body or the mind. We have proven that you can heal any dysfunction of the mind or body *if you want to.*

Everyone will say they want to be healed. But unfortunately, many do not want to confront the fear of change or give up the mileage they're getting out of their dysfunction or disease. If you want to be taken care of and you have created the dysfunction to achieve that end, any progress in healing will take major transformation to your belief system. Most people who are stuck in their illusion will deny that they're holding themselves back. It's obvious to me when a client is stuck or doesn't want to move past the blocks. The breakdown is in the will and desire to take responsibility to overcome the adversity, and there's little use in working with them. In fact, clients may get mad with you for trying to push your truth on them. If their illusion is their truth, then your view is an illusion to them. It is almost impossible to change a person's illusion, and we cannot instill the will to change. Clients must choose to claim their personal power. In fact, if I do point out their denial, they will cling to the addiction even harder. Many times, I will lose them as clients or friends because they will see me as a self-righteous meddler.

With biofeedback, the Subconscious Mind will respond to any question and validate the response so well that we can pinpoint the exact date of the traumatic incident and the client's age at the time. With appropriate questioning, we can locate any blocked trauma in a client's life. Since we are working directly with the Subconscious Mind, the Middle Self cannot block or resist. We can even watch the biofeedback response as the trauma/pattern is released.

Those who are skeptical that N/CR can locate the actual programs can graphically watch the release on the biofeedback instrument. This is a new adjunct to counseling which has a far-reaching effect for clients not getting results from counseling. It is an effective tool for use in healing, because we can quickly get to any base cause.

Biofeedback is also an excellent tool to recognize how much control your Middle Self has over you. The Middle Self cannot block the information. You can begin a dialogue with your Middle Self and make friends with it. By cutting through its defenses, you let it know where it tries to control. This is one of the few ways you can work on yourself. You can process yourself in an effective manner when you learn how to use the instruments. We feel this is the next step on the path to personal transformation and self-healing.

Over the past seven years, I have become familiar with how the mind responds/reacts to biofeedback. I have developed a method to dialogue with the Middle Self that will get it to release its control and cooperate with you. It is very easy to recognize when the Middle Self is blocking; the withholds, denials and illusions are obvious, and we know when we have released the core issue. The client can watch his or her temperature go down on resistance and up on acceptance.

Once I was asking a client a series of questions, and we saw the resistance building as body temperature started to drop. The closer I got to the core issue, the more it dropped. We finally had to stop the session because the client was getting nauseated when his temperature dropped from 98.6 to 72 degrees even though the outside temperature was about 80 degrees.

When a denial becomes a denial-of-denial, the results are dramatic. Middle Self resists and the client goes along with it, which creates fear that leads to stomach upset and nausea. This client was a major controller in the family and didn't want to admit it; it was everyone else's problem. *They* had the relationship problems and the discipline problems with the children. It was no surprise that I never saw that client again. This happens quite often when one gets face-to-face with a denial-of-denial.

Chapter 13

My Journey Into Healing

As a healing researcher since 1978, I use myself as my own laboratory to try new concepts. For the first seven years, being unable to find any alternative therapy that would totally relieve the pain in my body, I believed the doctors' prognosis that I would have to live with the pain for the rest of my life, and if it became unbearable, take painkillers. Their final prognosis was that my spine would deteriorate to the point that my muscles could no longer support my weight and I would be confined to a wheelchair. *I proved their prognosis totally false. The battle with your body can be won.*

I have achieved that end without surgery or drugs. Let's say that doctors are not wrong; they can only understand what their training and research gives them. Since few doctors do research, their education ends when they graduate from medical school. I was not willing to accept the doctors' diagnosis and went beyond what the linear mind could comprehend. If my body could create this pain, something was making it do this and I wanted to know what. However, I had no idea how I would accomplish this. But, "When the student is ready, the teacher will appear."

In a 1978 workshop, Ronald Beesley asked any participants who had severe pain or a major dysfunction affecting their life to submit a written description and he would select six people to use as demonstrators. One of those was me, and miraculously, for the first time in 17 years, I was pain-free after 20 minutes. However, it only lasted for a few days.

One of Beesley's students, Reg Newbon, had an office 3½ hours from my home, and I committed to a session every other week. I went to him for about two years for treatments.

Reg Newbon's treatment revealed many of the causes for my pain. He used hands-on, touching the various points on the body which he said held the imprint of the experience that caused the pain. By holding the point, he was able release the charge held in that location. By massaging along each side of the spine, pushing into the center of the spine from both sides. He also cleared the etheric fields and the chakras. I was so impressed by the process that I attended three one-week workshops—an important stepping stone in my path.

The problem was that the pain would return if I did not keep to the schedule. Why, I wondered, did the pain keep coming back?

I started going to the hot springs in nearby Calistoga in the Napa Valley, and had a deep tissue massage from Frank Hughes, the owner of Nance's Hot Springs. Going far beyond just a relaxing experience, his technique is more manipulation of the muscles and bones similar to osteopathy. When I started out, I had a double "S" curve in my spine, and had shrunk a full inch in height between ages 30 and 40. The vertebrae were so tight that he could not move them by himself and needed an assistant to hold me down as he tried to relax the muscles. It was painful, but my posture slowly returned.

I explored other alternative therapies to supplement Frank's work, but few people were willing to use the necessary force. I was frustrated because most physical therapists claimed they could heal me, but none did; the pain always returned. In hindsight, my expectations may have been too high; the practitioners were doing the best they could, but their best wasn't good enough. *I wanted the pain gone.*

In 1978, I became involved in *A Course In Miracles*, but after the first five lessons, I found it too intense and threatening, and stopped reading. Later that year, I attended a seminar in San Diego—the Mandala Conference, at which Jampolsky presented a workshop—and was so enthused that I started going to his weekly groups.

I was amazed at the energy in the group some nights; all we did was hold hands in a circle asking for help, and people would be healed on the spot.

I also met Paul Solomon at that same seminar, and three months later, got a call out of the blue: "Paul is holding a workshop today in Palo Alto and you're supposed to be there, but we forgot to let you know. The introductory lecture was last night, but you can attend the first day of the workshop for ten dollars. Sorry about the short notice." After that message, how could I not go?

The workshop was more than I expected, and changed my life forever. It was being repeated the next weekend, and I cancelled my plans so that I could attend. I became deeply involved with Solomon's work, almost to the point of addiction. I attended every West Coast event for the next ten years, including a one-week and a two-week residential workshop. In 1982, I even attended a two-week teacher training course in Virginia Beach.

The most memorable aspect of his work was what he called the "X-Factor in Healing"—the need to integrate all levels of body/mind and spirit to cause healing to take place, and the need for clear and focused intention to the purpose of healing. He talked about spontaneous healing miracles in which clients were brought to an intention that was so complete that they let go of fear and anger, resulting in instantaneous healing. This has happened to me a few times with clients.

The next most important ingredient, he said, is unconditional love. When that is present, miracles also happen. My experience with clients since has shown me that healers must have their own "love issues" resolved and be coming from 100 percent unconditional self-love. Then their clients will have amazing results.

When clients can feel the practitioner's love coming to them with no withholds or needs attached, healing miracles can take place. The practitioner must be able to project this caring to the point that more than 50 percent is directed towards the client. To me, this is the critical factor in healing. How could I do love-based work if I did not know what love is?

With Paul's guidance in mind, I set out to understand love. No one in my family had known what love was, let alone demonstrate unconditional love. My parents gave me material things and called it love, but there were always strings attached. There was no love in their childhood either, so they were doing the best they knew how.

My first task, then, was to recognize the love deficiency in my life, so I started to attend workshops that involved vulnerability and support, beginning with a week-long workshop with Paul Solomon. When I saw men hugging, all manner of fears came up and my first impulse was to leave. My family had been judgmental, with no intimacy, so all my childhood programs were challenged. However, I stuck it out, and when I went home, the first thing I did was tell my wife Susie that I loved her. Up until then, she'd had to dig it out of me. For some reason, even saying the word "love" scared me.

A surprised Susie said, "Can I attend one of those workshops? I'd like to get some of what you got." We both attended the next workshop and it totally changed our relationship. We realized that for thirteen years, we had simply been living in the same house.

The more I dug into what causes healing to happen, the more I wondered what drove my body back into pain between my bi-weekly treatments. I realized that although they both had the same end result in mind and both worked to release pain, Reg Newbon and Frank Hughes were coming from opposite ends of the spectrum— Reg from a purely spiritual orientation, and Frank from the position that if you press hard enough on the body's trigger points and adjust the muscles, the tension will release. Frank was having more success, so I stopped going to Reg. But I knew there had to be more than weekly treatments. Why were my muscles tightening up all the time?

Between 1977 and 1981, the more I studied with Paul Solomon along with my training for a Masters degree in Psychology, I realized that the emotional component of dysfunction needed to be understood. But no teachers were talking about how to apply psychological principles to pain in the body (only in the late 1990s have people have become more aware of somatic (body/mind) oriented therapy). So, I decided to apply all the guidance that my teachers offered, plus some new directions. I attended seminars on Chinese and Tibetan Medicine at U.C. Berkeley, and a workshop on Homeopathy with George Vithoulkas. He looked at a person as an integrated unit in which the body as a manifestation of personality, thoughts, emotions and sensations. This was the right direction, but the training was too long and arduous. I tried Ayurveda with the same results; going through all the processes to find the cause, let alone treat it, would take many years.

In April of 1979, I attended Paul Solomon's two-week live-in seminar on Advanced Inner Light Conscious. It was a real eye-opener; on the third day, I started feeling very cold and as soon as the session started, I turned white as a sheet and passed out. When I came to at the break, I was unaware that I'd passed out and denied it. When the session resumed 15 minutes later, I passed out again. When I finally came to at the end of the session, I felt as though I'd been hit by a truck and went to bed. The following morning, I could barely move. I skipped breakfast and finally got to the morning session late. All I wanted to do was go home. Something in me was extremely scared and did not want to be there. In fact, ten other people left over the next two weeks, but I'd paid my money and was determined to finish the course no matter how much my body/mind resisted.

One of the instructors agreed to work with me to find out what was going on. We found that every concept I held about who I was felt threatened. The concentrated energy of being with those people and the intensity of the work was forcing my whole being to change all of its beliefs. My fragile reality was threatened. For example, I didn't realize until then that I was a control addict and, by today's standards, a counter-dependent.

The following days were a little easier, but I was still on edge. I got rebuked for talking too much and monopolizing conversations. More processing revealed that I felt accepted if people would let me control the conversation. That workshop taught me many painful lessons around acceptance and validation. Needless to say, I came out of it a very different person. However, I was addicted to such high-intensity workshops, and attended three more. I just couldn't seem to satisfy my thirst for a new life, and couldn't understand why others did not have the same drive.

In 1982, we settled a legal action that freed up some funds, and my family and I spent almost four months traveling around the U.S. This gave me time to take stock. With five people confined in an RV, we were able to work out and practice what we had learned. By the end of the trip, I understood why my pain always returned. It was caused by resurfacing beliefs and programs that were driving my life. Frank would release the pent-up energy by working my trigger points, my body and muscles would relax, healing would seem to have happened, but the driving force was still there. Over the following days, the stress and tension of daily life would rebuild, and the muscles would tighten up again.

Suddenly, in 1982, my whole reality shifted when I saw clearly how programs were driving my life. Over the next two years, my understanding of this clarified. I was also doing much work on inner levels, communicating with the Source.

At a seminar on Hawaiian Huna work, someone asked me to help his daughter, who suffered from prism vision. I discovered that it was a genetic condition caused by a past life experience with her father. After the fourth session, the condition cleared up in two days and has never returned after 15 years. This was my introduction to miracle healing.

In 1984, I began to shift my whole practice to hands-on work. I lost those clients who simply wanted a therapist to hold their hand and commiserate about how bad their life was. I determined to work only with clients who demonstrated progress in each session.

My first experience with this new integrated process was with a male client who was having trouble dealing with women. He had lost two jobs from this fear and was about to get fired for missing work. I focused on his situation and went directly to the problem at hand, but still could not help clear his fear of women. I asked him lie down on my massage table, and found a large painful lump on his back near his left shoulder blade. I put my hand on it and an affirmation came from my inner self: "I know that my mother treated me badly, and I felt rejected and abandoned by her. I recognize she was doing the best she could and I accept that now. I realize she did not know the effect she was having on me. I am loving and forgiving her now, unconditionally."

Immediately, the lump and the pain disappeared completely. Not only that, he was able to return to work. Of course, clearing one program brought up many more, but after many sessions, we had cleared the whole situation.

This experience confirmed my decision to abandon talk therapy because it was only marginally effective. I realized I had discovered why my own pain returned after each release—it was the programming! As I explored this further, I discovered it was the reprogramming by affirmations that released the pain. I also realized that I could not do the reprogramming for my clients. I could develop the program for them, but they themselves had to delete the old program and install the new one. The big "ah-ha" for me was that in saying the affirmation for the client to repeat, I was reprogramming myself at the same time. During the next five years, I was able to cause my own healing by working with my clients.

Many of my colleagues were suspicious of what I was doing. Some resented my success, while others referred clients to me when they ran into immovable blocks. As word spread of my results, my client list grew quickly, and my back pain started releasing because I was able to include myself into the therapy process along with clients who had similar programs and patterns to mine. Over the next four years, I cleared much of my pain. By stating the affirmations for the clients to repeat, I was helped almost as much as they were.

My next miracle came shortly after I began my body-based therapy. I was giving a weekly lecture, and an attendee asked, "Can you do something about back pain that was created by surgery? I understand your problem is similar to mine, but the difference is that the surgery was not successful."

She had four vertebrae tied together with stainless steel wire. Because her back would not fuse after the first surgery, the doctors removed the discs and wired the vertebrae up to force them to fuse. The pain was so intense that she was on the verge of suicide. She ended her question with, "I want you to heal me."

Until then, I called myself a healer, so my response surprised even me. "I can't heal you; only you can heal you. I just show you the way."

I didn't know what to think when, after our session, she called to say that the pain had gone and she would come back next week. When we went into the process, we found that most of her problems were past-life, tied in with her parents in this life, both of whom totally rejected her. In fact, they had not wanted any children, so she was rejected before birth. I discovered that all her back problems were caused by self-rejection. If she was not wanted by her parents, so why would anyone want her? She had so many "I'm not alright" programs attached to the self-rejection that they had actually been eating away her vertebrae and discs.

She set another appointment but later called to cancel. She had been in a car accident and needed X-rays to see if she had any injuries. She later called me, bursting with excitement, saying, "Do you believe in miracles? The latest X-rays showed that the wire is gone and all the discs are back, perfect, as well as the vertebrae. What do you make of that?"

Removed discs grown back? Wire disappeared? Yes, it was a miracle, but at the time, I had no idea how it happened. I now know that this happens all the time with N/CR. The infinite power of the mind can heal immediately if you are committed to healing.

As I continued working with the process, I was making great progress with my clients but there was nobody to work on me. In September, 1987, Chris Issel asked me to teach a workshop on the process if she could get a group together. Chris became so proficient in N/CR that we began trading. My progress to be pain free quickly became a reality. At this point, N/CR, made a major leap; I was now on the road, speaking at bookstores and giving lectures and workshops all over California.

In 1989, I met Mike Hammer, and he learned N/CR as if he already knew it. I needed a workshop co-presenter and Mike was a perfect match for me. We learned much during our three years together, and by trading sessions with Mike, I finally became pain-free after 30 years.

With all the new practitioners trained in NCR, my horizons rapidly opened up. My body was now really talking to me. Odd pains surfaced, but in different places on my body. I had plenty of help in understanding the causes and releasing the pain.

From 1991 to 1996, the information floodgates opened. I had a steady stream of partners with whom I could do research. We found how to release pain anytime it appears by looking for the lesson or the cellular memory that's talking. Many times, it's a Middle Self fear-based interpretation that has no value. In an effort to protect us, Middle Self will set up what it thinks is a valid reaction. This requires us to take it to task over making decisions about our health and direction without our permission.

At one point, a friend asked me if I'd worked out all of my mother issues. I said yes, because I'd been working on them for over ten years. That really sparked a reaction that brought up issues that I had no idea were still active, such as my unwillingness to tell the truth, especially to my mother. Once I saw my habit of telling people what they wanted to hear so I would not get rejected, my left shoulder locked up so badly that I needed pain killers for the first time in over 20 years. Over the next week, eight people worked on me for a total of 14 hours to clear the old programs. This opened a whole new area in N/CR: denial. We bury issues we don't want to deal with if they are too painful or fearful to handle.

New areas keep opening up all the time. For example, in July, 1996, I mysteriously started to lose my hearing, and by December, I was stone-deaf. Refusing to accept that any dysfunction is final, I continued giving lectures and workshops, and by September, 1997, with the help of Bernard Eakes, I had recovered my hearing completely, only to lose it again in December. We located the programs and I recovered it again, but in July,

1998, I again partially lost it. As of Spring 1999, I have recovered the hearing in my left ear, but it continues to come and go as more programs and sub-personalities surface. Each occurrence has been due to fear: of presenting the N/CR concepts and my new devices from electronic medical research, and of publishing my books. A deep fear program that people will not be interested in the books and they will not sell has been a stumbling block for many years. I would sit down at my computer to work on a book and pass out as the survival-oriented programs and beliefs in Middle Self tried to prevent me from writing in case I made a fool out of myself. However, once I knew what was happening, I could deal with the sub-personalities responsible.

As of reprinting this book in September 2001, I have not had any reoccurrence of deafness as I finally made it over the hill in my own alrightness. After over 20 years of trying to prove my concepts, I realized that I do not have do this anymore; I do not have to prove anything. The concepts can stand alone in world of alternative healing, as proven by books being sold in many countries around the world. It is only a start but acceptance is now building, and we receive calls from within the U.S. and Canada, plus many countries around the world asking for information about our work and when we plan to be in the caller's country. Ironically, while I appreciate the validation, I no longer need it.

To understand why we separate from self, we must reconstruct our childhood. The reason psychotherapy does not get to the cause is that it cannot reveal how our childhood programming affected us the way it did since we seldom accurately remember our childhood experiences. Therapists can only work with what clients tell them, and most of the time, clients describe the results of their feeling about an incident in their life, which is the result of the programming. They don't understand the programming but they are reacting to it.

This has to do with how we react to a stimulus before us. Two twins can react totally differently to their parents even though the parents claim they treated the twins exactly the same. As a therapist, because I was clairvoyant, I was able to actually read the program files and describe them to my clients. However, I wasn't able to reprogram the mind's files at the time, but I now have the tools to do exactly that.

A good example of this is the following childhood experience. In the 1940s, school teachers favored right-handed children and looked down on left-handed children as if they had something wrong with them. I was ambidextrous but favored my left hand. Thinking they were helping me, my teachers forced me to use my right hand. The result was total dysfunction in my bicameral brain interpretation. Added to this was the stress of my mother leaving the family home. The fragmentation caused by feeling that I had to please the teacher destroyed my self-worth, and I became totally dyslexic, unable to read or write. Whatever I wrote came out backwards, and the teacher had to hold the paper up to a mirror. When I read aloud, the words were reversed and sounded like some code language.

Instead of understanding the problem the teachers had caused, they classified me as "learning disabled." By adulthood, I did not even know this had happened to me because I was suppressing it to the point of denial-of-denial. After clearing this incident, my residual dyslexia with numbers disappeared and I can now speed-read without any problems.

It is difficult for men to show emotion or express their feelings if it shows them as vulnerable. I broke this barrier when I realized that sub-personalities were causing me to act with a macho male attitude of having to be strong, never showing emotions, and always having to be right. These are what one would call Ego. When we understood Ego and realized what was creating these personality self-traits, I was able to overcome it and allow myself to become open and vulnerable. When this happened, I realized that I became more accepted and trusted.

One of the major breakthroughs came with the movie *Field Of Dreams*, which brought up so much emotion that my wife, Susie, took almost a half hour to process it out. I realized that I had not cleared with my father before he died. He was my champion, yet I did not know it since my mother had verbally beaten him up so badly that one day he just walked out and died. I knew at the time (1976) that I had to do something the day before he passed on, but I did not know what it was.

It was very disturbing to me because I had helped heal him from four life-threatening illnesses. The doctors gave him three months to live after they found pancreatic cancer, but he lived for many years after the cancer was healed. Until I saw this movie, I had stuffed all my feelings, but they all came pouring out at once. One of the most troubling feelings was that my son had been deprived of his grandfather, who had adored him. They had a bond that was building a supportive relationship, which my son missed for a long time.

When I would work with a client who had the same experience, or I would describe my experience in a lecture, emotions would start and tears would flow. It did not seem to bother me anymore and actually drew people in more when they saw that I could be vulnerable in front of them and allow my feelings to surface.

A client recently brought Wayne Dyers new tape set, *There is a Spiritual Solution To Every Problem,* to a session and insisted I listen to it. He said, "It sounds like you're talking to me in a different voice. This is what you've been saying for fifteen years. Why is it that Wayne Dyer gets an audience and you don't seem to get the exposure?"

I asked him, "How many of Wayne's books have you read?"

"All of them," he replied.

My response was, "Well, what does that tell you? He has been writing books and speaking to audiences for over twenty-five years. My books have only been in stores for three years. You don't get recognition until you get books published."

At that, he said, "I guess your time is coming then."

As I was revising this book and listening to the tapes, some of the stories and anecdotes brought up many tears and emotions. When these emotions come up, I realize that denial-of-denial programs are surfacing. I had not dealt with these issues. The tapes are catalysts and they will always bring up suppressed files. We must be willing to deal with these files when they come up as they are limiting our enlightenment and evolvement. Sometimes in sessions, I will have an emotional reaction when the same issues surface for clients that I have not worked out. So we both have the chance to get our feelings out and clear them. Some therapists find this embarrassing because they do not feel they are the strong leaders they should be. However, the result of their avoidance attitude puts clients in a hard place to deal with.

There is much more to my journey on this path, which appears in my book *Becoming A Spiritual Being In A Physical Body*.

Chapter 14

Typical Cases

When I began this work in 1978 I was not aware of the potential of my discoveries. I was amazed that all I had to do was put my hands in the right places, and the acupuncture points I touched on the body acted as an extension of my mind. As if I was watching a video, I saw the very experience that the client was talking about. Quite often, my own experience would merge with the client's experience I was seeing.

To speed up the process, I asked clients, before they came to me, to list the issues with which they wanted to work, and not surprisingly, those issues were exactly what would come up in session. And even though we'd use the very same acupuncture points in subsequent sessions, different issues would come up, as if we were pealing an onion

I carefully documented clients' cases to help us better learn about the mind and the dynamics it operated from. Actual names are not given to protect client confidentiality. If any reader would like to contact clients directly, I will ask them if they wish to talk about their case and have that client contact the reader.

Many times, all I do is get the program going and if the client is committed, processing will continue and self-healing take place. In some cases, we have to work an issue through each week over time. The most important part of the therapy seems to be the desire to let go of the dysfunction and take a new path. If clients are getting mileage out of a dysfunction, I can't do much for them.

It is important to understand that the key to healing is your ability to let go of the illusion that is blocking healing. As you will see in these examples, time to heal is not related to the severity of the dysfunction. Many times, a severe dysfunction will change in minutes, yet others may take years. The following cases discuss the basic dysfunctional program and how it was handled. The most important point to keep in mind is: How many years did it take to create all the programs? Do you expect to clear your life path in a few sessions?

We can remove the big stumbling blocks, but the programs and patterns that have been created from childhood traumas and fears have to be removed completely. It has taken me over 20 years to clear my path and I am not finished yet. But by understanding how the mind operates, along with the sub-personalities and their denial factors, we can dramatically curtail the time needed for recovery.

Case #1. At age six, the client was diagnosed with prism vision and today wears corrective glasses. Her school assumed she was learning disabled since she had to tilt her head at 45 degrees to see straight. The teachers' misreading of the situation effectively destroyed her self-esteem. Doctors declared it a genetic defect, and that nothing could be done other than wear corrective glasses. Although they work well, she is a semi-pro skater, and every time she jumps, her glasses fall off.

In four sessions, we identify the problem as a past-life issue with the father. Working with both the father and the daughter, we clear all their karmic contracts. By getting back to the base cause, we clear the path for the body to alter the DNA pattern and create perfect sight.

Case #2. The client has breast cancer that suddenly becomes radical. Because of the speed of growth, her doctors want to perform a mastectomy. She is a total vegetarian, no eggs or dairy, and has good relationships with her parents and her boyfriend. She has no problems at work. She runs 20 miles a week, does aerobics and rides a bicycle. A baffling case since all the outside things that cause cancer are not present.

As we work through her childhood, we find that her mother died of breast cancer when she was eight, as did two aunts. At the funeral, her family members were talking about how they must be very careful with their female children because this must run in the family. Her Middle Self accepted the belief and her Subconscious Mind programmed it in. When she turned 40, her mind had a program that she would get breast cancer, so it was manifested in her physical body like a time-bomb.

Once we release the program and the belief, we ask her mind to heal the cancer and erase all the programming. She has no reason to have cancer so it disappears in fifteen minutes. This is done with affirmations only. The client cancels all future doctor appointments.

Case #3. A client has severe pain. We find he was rejected by both parents due to mother's pregnancy prior to marriage. Also, the child was the wrong gender. In his mother/son relationship, he sought out a mother who would love him, and his neediness destroyed the relationship.

We release the pre-birth rejection with all its programs and then he forgives the parents. Clearing all the childhood self-rejection and the feeling of not being alright opens up new doors to balance. Forgiving involves working through all the childhood trauma and rejection up to the current relationship. The main change is his relationship with self. When that is cleared so that he can love himself, his life turns around and the pain simply vanishes.

Case #4. A female client asks why nothing works in her life. She has had many jobs but always seems to get laid off or fired. She has never had a successful relationship.

Severe pain along the spine indicates total self-rejection. We find she has no self-worth, that she feels her value is zero, so why would anyone want to have her as an employee?

In exploring her past, we find she was an unexpected "mistake" child who her mother tried to abort. She was treated like an intruder in the family. Her mother tried to delegate caring for her to her older siblings, who did not want to take it on, so even they rejected her.

We reclaim her self-worth and self-esteem by forgiving and understanding the parents and loving and forgiving her brothers and sisters. In clearing the rejection and abandonment, and re-claiming her personal power, we find that she has no program about self-love or receiving love. Once we reestablish balance in her life, she is able to get a good job and form a supportive rela-tionship.

Case #5. A 47-year-old woman has not had a stable relationship in her life. She has been married five times, and all ended with the husband cheating and having affairs. She does not love her-self and will not accept love from others. She is not functioning in her body, and her polarity is switched.

The first picture I see when looking for the points of pain is one of the father yelling at the mother, "You're giving this child all the attention. I don't get any attention anymore. This child is the center point in your life." The "adult-child" father feels re-jected because the mother has to take care of the child and the child competes with the father for the mother's love, while the mother has to straddle the fence to keep peace. The child cannot understand why she gets a lot of attention when the father is not there, but little when he's home.

Over about ten sessions, she reclaims her personal power, self-esteem, and self-worth.

Case #6. A client introduces me to his friend who stutters so badly that his neurology practice is almost empty. Who wants to see a stuttering neurologist? Apparently not many people.

With kinesiology, we find that he started stuttering 15 years ago when his house was burned down. In a past life, he burned a farmer's barn down in a fit of anger. The karmic lesson came back to roost. We clear the karmic contract and the stuttering stops. He is punishing himself for this lesson. He had already paid the price by losing his house but he is still punishing himself 15 years later.

He is so impressed he takes us to dinner, and in the restaurant, he begins to stutter again. I ask him, "Are you having doubts about what we've accomplished?"

He replies, "I'm having a hard time reconciling this situation. I have ten years of college in my specialty and you have no credentials as far as I can see. Yet, none of the neurologists or the speech therapists were able to accomplish anything, but you cleared it all in 20 minutes."

I ask him, "What's more important, credentials or the result? You can see and experience the result of stuttering and what it's done to your life, and now you're free of it."

He agrees, and we finish by repeating the affirmation and asking his Ego and Subconscious Mind to destroy the programs sabotaging his success and lock them up in the archives. That is the end of the stuttering for ever.

Case #7. A women is referred to me because she has flunked the teacher's credential test six times. She feels rejected by the system, and is willing to give up, accept her lot in life, and teach at a substandard level.

On checking, we find that her husband continually tells her she's no good at math so how can she expect to pass the test. She did have problems with math in school, but her field has no math in it so that's not the problem. She has a program about giving her power to authority figures. Her husband is an attorney, and she gives her power away to him. (As children, this program is meant to give respect to our parents and obey them, but as adults, it has no value.) We identify her challenge as stopping giving her power away to authority figures.

We release the belief and the program about not being good at math and reinforce her personal power by erasing the authority figure program. We write new scripts to take her power back and know that she can pass the test effortlessly, which she does so on the next try, passing in the 92nd percentile. (In the past, she could not even finish the test in the allotted time.)

What is the difference? Her self-worth and her self-esteem have been recovered. She now sees herself as all right, as a person who has innate value. The "system" had nothing to do with rejecting her; it was her self-rejection and lack of perceivd value that caused her failure, as with most people.

Case #8. A client labels her symptoms as Chronic Fatigue Syndrome. On evaluation, I find she's telling herself that she is "sick and tired of this and that" all the time. She is really backing out of life and does not want to participate. All her life, she has taken care of others. Her Middle Self accepts the "sick and tired" statements. Coupled with the caretaker personality, her Ego and Middle Self listen to her constantly telling herself she should stop, so they step in to help as best they can.

When I bring this up to her, she is amazed to learn that our thoughts have power. We release the program about being sick and tired and reclaim her power to say "no" when people impose on her. The fatigue disappears.

Case #9. A client has severe bursitis, and in working with him, I discover in me a lot of suppressed anger towards my mother. I do not want to accept it, but I find that I have my mother on a pedestal: "You have to respect and accept mothers unconditionally." I uncover denial, but don't know how to handle it at the time.

As we struggle through over 14 hours of work with eight different practitioners, my left shoulder locks up. My shoulder pain is excruciating, as though a knife has been stuck in my shoulder. After a very painful week, we finally clear it. Now we can walk throughout the same process in a session or two.

Symptoms such as this are about saying how we feel and speaking our truth. Telling people what they want to hear rather than saying what you want to say will only intensify the condition. Most people try to blame it on a pulled muscle.

I have found the pain can be released as soon as we release the feeling of not being alright, and can reclaim our personal power so that we can speak our truth. Once we write a new script, the pain goes away. The lesson is to take our power back and release ourselves from the fear of rejection.

Why the mind chooses a particular dysfunction is unknown. Two people may be in the same situation but manifest different dysfunctions, depending on the core issue. For example, the neurological dysfunction of Multiple Sclerosis (MS), Lou Gehrig Disease (ALS), Muscular Dystrophy (MD) and Parkinson's Disease all operate from the same basic program, yet exhibit different symptoms. My work with many people with these conditions has met with marginal success. Clients want to escape something in their life path, but if they are willing to face what they are running away from, we can release and heal it. Many times, they are trying to force someone to take care of them, usually stemming from childhood attempts to get recognition by someone.

Neurological dysfunction presents some of the most difficult cases to deal with, as clients are usually in denial of their anger. They are getting a lot of satisfaction for their resentment, and the sub-personalities want to hold on to the condition because it provides a means of controlling others.

Case #10. With an MS client, we begin with looking at the childhood programs that are similar to those held by many rejected children. Feeling unacknowledged at school and not appreciated for his work, he became a super-student, trying to impress his parents that he had value. Although he graduated from college at the top of his class, it seemed that nobody would validate his accomplishments. After a few failures in business, he began to develop MS symptoms, and they progressed to the point where he became wheelchair-bound.

When I meet him, he is making a commitment to recover. A controlling sub-personality is running his life and forcing people to take care of him. In this way, his mind's interpretation is that he is finally getting acknowledged.

After many sessions, we get him back on his feet and functioning. His Middle Self and Ego are intent on getting this end result and they don't care how they do it. When he reclaims his power and regains control over his life, he recovers completely.

Case #11. At one of my lectures, a very intelligent woman asks me about MS. Apparently, brain scans and MRI showed lesions on her brain that indicate MS. She is an instructor at a college, but has become so debilitated she lost her job, which caused a rapid downturn in her health. She can no longer drive a car and is considered legally blind. She is losing motor control of her legs and arms. She is also trying to escape an abusive husband who is not functioning rationally. She is finally able to break free when he ends up the hospital and almost dies.

When we look at her situation, we also find a very abusive childhood. I work with her over a two-year period and we recover her eyesight so that she can drive a car and walk again. At this point, she is recovering slowly.

Case #12. Another MS client drives over five hours to see me. In two sessions, we clear the total disease syndrome and she returns to perfectly normal health. Her base causes were the same as all the others, but the difference is that she is willing to let the past go and release herself from blaming anyone. When she accepts that she created the MS to get a desired result, she is able to break the disease syndrome completely. (This is the hardest syndrome to break down and get a person to reclaim their personal power.)

Case #13. When a client was not validated for his ability, he became a book worm to prove that he could be someone. He graduated from UC Berkeley, *magna cum laud*, but the only problem was that he cut himself off from everybody and everything in his life to succeed.

He joined a group led by a guru who insisted that his followers had to do everything his way. This matched his program because he wanted someone to run his life for him. He met his wife in this group, and she was very controlling. This also served his need to be validated. He worked for a bank and had good performance reviews, so he was promoted, but this validation came from the outside, and not from within, so was worthless.

A week after he started his new job, he had a grand mal seizure at work and was taken to the hospital. He also had his driver's license revoked so his wife has to drive him to work and to my appointment.

He is able to recognize the program, release the pattern, and reclaim his personal power, but once he does, he starts to have relationship problems. His wife objects to him taking his power back because she enjoys their "mother/son" relationship as it was. The more he tries to regain control of his life, the more angry she gets, and eventually divorces him. At this latest rejection, down he goes and has to have friends drive him to the appointments. We finally get him back on his feet so he can function once more.

Case #14. A women comes to me because she has just lost her job for the sixteenth time and has been through a divorce from her fifth husband, all five of whom parallel her father's behavior. She is looking for a "father" who will love and validate her, and faces the timeworn challenge of standing up, taking her power back and validating herself.

Her problems started when she was three days old, and lying in the hospital bed with her mother. Her father walked in and began to berate the mother for almost dying in childbirth and having a fourth child that they could not afford. He was irate that she had to stay in the hospital for another week under observation.

I witness the dialogue coming directly from her Subconscious Mind, yet she has no knowledge of this incident at all. When she goes to her mother with this information, her mother denies it.

When we get her strong enough to confront her parents, she tells them that what they want to believe does not make any difference, and that she has released their lies, and feels great. She tells them she has forgiven them and that she loves them for who they are. They all break down and, in a "happily ever after" outcome, talk the situation out.

She soon finds a great relationship and new job that's better than the last one she lost. Six months later, she calls to tell me she is now married and life is beautiful. All this took only six sessions.

Case #15. In 1986, a female client has the most interesting disease I have ever seen, breast cancer for the third time. However, she'd had cancer twice and had both breasts removed at different times. This time, the tumor is attached to the ribcage. I ask her, "Are you sure you want to live?"

Although she says "Yes," I find that she is in denial. Even though we release her "I want to die" program, it's back the following week. In her Middle Self, we find a program about wanting to die because she cannot control her husband (of which she is in total denial). We make peace with her attitude about her husband, and the "I want to die" program is gone.

Next, I ask her to put her cancer in my hand. She refuses, saying she doesn't want me to get cancer. I assure her that getting her cancer is not in my karmic pattern. She lets go of the cancer, and the force of it knocks me to the floor. That is my first experience of the power of vector disease energy when it lets go. (Now, I sit down when doing that treatment.)

I have encountered at least ten clients with the desire to die rather than deal with a personal confrontation. In the following three cases, I was unable to redirect the "I want to die" program.

Case #16. My father has four life threatening diseases, including pancreatic cancer. The doctor has given him three months to live. He tries chemotherapy but finds it too painful and upsetting, so he follows my suggestions and, with the help of a sympathetic doctor, it is gone in six months. (In this country, cancer is big money, and the medical profession, FDA, and the medical boards conspired to run the doctor out of California and the U.S. He is very successful at treating cancer with alternative methods, and the vested interests wanted him out of business.)

Four years later, my father is totally clear of cancer, but needs an operation for an obstructed intestine. When he dies about a year and a half later, the hospital tries to list his death as cancer, so I force them to perform an autopsy and they find no cancer at all, so they list his death as lung congestion. In truth, he left because he did not want to confront my mother. She is a master controller and he has given his power away to her. He gave up rather than follow his own desire to move near us to be close to his grandson. He died at 76 and mother lived to 94. When she decided to go, within 24 hours, she was gone

Case #17. A client who has been doing very well goes into decline when her husband leaves her alone for two weeks. He has taken elk-hunting trips for many years without any ill effects; the difference now is that she wants to hire a person to clean the house once or twice a week. The husband objects and says that because he is now retired, he will help her. However, he is unwilling to clean the way she wants, and this blows up into a major conflict in their relationship. When he leaves for his trip, she feels overwhelmed and stops coming to me. When he returns, he does not support her desire to resume treatments with me.

About six months later, he calls to tell me that his wife wants to see me but can't leave the house. I make the house call and find her withered away and barely able to talk. I give her the last rites, help her forgive herself for allowing this to happen, and give her permission to leave. I tell the husband that she will be gone in less than 24 hours. He calls me the following morning to confirm that she died during the night.

Case #18. Recommended by a friend, a man with colon cancer comes to see me. He and his wife are very wealthy and own a multimillion dollar business. The wife is a workaholic and wants her husband to be the same.

Colon cancer is invariably caused by repressed anger, so that's where we start. Over time, I'd think we've cleared it all but am unaware of active sub-personality problems. He starts taking time off in the morning to play handball, which infuriates his wife. He convinces her to see me, but all she does is complain about how lazy her husband is. For some reason, that marks the beginning of the end. He just starts withering away, with no real definable illness. He has many sessions with me, for which they pay well, but I am unable to pull him out of his downward spiral. He hangs on for a long time even though I give him permission to leave. What he wants is the love and attention that he never received from his mother or his wife. When he finally dies, I tell his wife why, but she totally denies any part in his death and criticizes me for my opinion.

Case #19. Another colon cancer client with a controlling workaholic wife comes to me after surgery in the hope that I can find the cause so it will not reoccur. We clear all the usual causes for the cancer, but he chooses another means of death in order to escape his wife's control. He is completely unable to stand up to her and take his power back, and I am unable to stop him from creating his own death.

He is very wealthy and she is angry that he is not putting in the hours that she wants him devote to the business. In fact, she gets mad at me for recommending that he take time for recreation and exercise. Unable to digest food, he starts to lose weight and falls back.

Since there seems nothing I can do, I suggest that they go to a clinic in Mexico. The doctors at the clinic say they cannot do anything either because he no longer wants to live and is not making any progress. I spend many hours with him trying to turn him around, but his wife has such control over him that I am unable to do so. He is suffering so I suggest to his wife that she give him permission to die. She does and he is gone the next morning. However, since I discovered how to defuse the "I want to die" program, I haven't lost another client.

Case #20. At a conference, a man asks me if I've had much luck with diabetes, a condition from which he almost died a year earlier. His eyesight is deteriorating, and his body is covered with large red splotches and bruises. His blood-sugar level is 410 (normal is 150), and he has to take insulin twice a day.

In about an hour, we have cleared all the causes. I meet him six weeks later, and he tells me that his doctor confirms that he no longer has diabetes. All the symptoms have cleared, including the bruises and red ulcerated spots on his legs. I compliment him on his commitment, and tell him that if a person is as committed as he is, it works every time. Miracles are in your control and you create them.

Case #21. Many clients suffer from sciatic nerve pain, and I have found that it is invariably connected with an "I'm not all right" program, one of the most prevalent I see. In my case, sciatic nerve pain crippled me almost to the point that at times I couldn't walk. It is almost always rooted in pre-birth rejection which keeps on building from many other situations throughout life. Almost every client has between ten and several hundred programs locked in many body locations besides the sciatic nerves in the legs. Many clients cannot sit for more than an hour or so without needing to walk around for a few minutes. In addition to the pain, this rules out lengthy auto trips.

In all cases, this program stems from feeling rejected and abandoned as a child, and is compounded by rejection before birth. The parents' actual treatment of the child is not always the problem, but the child's perception of how it is treated. They can give a child all the right material comforts and educational opportunities, yet a child may still feel unloved and rejected. It is the personal touch and sense of love and acceptance that is required. Another child can grow up in what would be considered a deprived family, and be showered with far more love, support and encouragement to succeed in life than the pampered child.

Case #22. A new client comes to me because he cannot hold his head up without a brace. Take the brace off and his head falls down and rests on his shoulder. He has no strength in his neck muscles at all and is unable to work. Also, he is controlling of his wife. Neck pain is caused by not wanting to take responsibility for one's life. When I tell him that if we clear up his dysfunction, he will have to go back to work and must work at not controlling his wife, he refuses to continue the session.

Case #23. A man comes to one of my lectures on the recommendation of his friend. He knows nothing about alternative healing or personal transformation, but starts attending my weekly lectures, and even comes for a session before the lecture, during which we start breaking down problems from his childhood. One day, he says, "I want to work on my eyesight. You say that if a person wants to see their life clearly, they can regenerate their eyes. I'm ready for that."

We begin working on the reason why his eyes have deteriorated, and soon his eyes begin to clear up. One day, he announces that he is able to read without his glasses. A year later, he tells me, "I can see so well now that I don't even carry my glasses around any more."

This has happened to many people. There is only one catch—seeing your life clearly takes great commitment because this is where denials really come into play.

Case #24. A client has serious breathing problems, yet the doctors cannot discover why. As I probe the area where she says it hurts, I find a very interesting program: fear of vulnerability and conditional acceptance. The programs are along the edge of the last rib from the side all the way to the center. When we clear all the programs, she can breathe normally.

Case #25. A man comes to my lecture with the intent of having me clear a diarrhea problem. He has to take the pills every three to four hours to keep it in control. His doctor (authority figure) has warned him that diarrhea is one of the side effects of the heart medicine he is taking. He stops the heart medication and uses chelation therapy instead, but, the diarrhea continues.

We release the doctor's proclamation and instructions in twenty minutes; the diarrhea stops immediately. If the program is a belief and not a reality, then it can be released with a simple affirmation.

Case #26. A woman client has the same back pain problem that I did. About twice a year, she has to go to the hospital and get an injection of muscle relaxant.

Middle back pain can cause major problems. Self-rejection will cause the muscles alongside the spine to contract. I got to the point where I could not lift more then ten pounds without throwing my back out. The muscles would go into spasm and I could not move. The doctors wanted me in the hospital for traction to stretch it out, but I refused their kind offer. Today, with the help of the people who learned N/CR, my back is normal. We cleared the client's problem in about five sessions.

Case #27. At one of my lectures, a concert cello player asks about scalaraderma, but I have not heard of the condition. We set up a session so that we can explore the cause.

Apparently, her mother had forced her, as a child, to play the violin for three to six hours a day to get ready for a recital. Having had enough abuse, she quit playing after the recital. Eight years later, her high school orchestra needed a cello player so she volunteered. After high school, she continued with the cello and joined the Palo Alto Symphony Orchestra, but her mother refused to attend any of the concerts, triggering a sense of rejection. Many years later, her local Unity Church asked her to give a solo performance, for which she got a standing ovation. Her mother, however, still refused to attend.

Shortly after this, she contracted scalaraderma. There is no known cure, and it's just a matter of time until the body simply ceases to function. The cause is an inability to handle her audiences' unconditional acceptance. In three sessions, we clear the causes and the disease disappears.

Case #28. My son believes totally in the N/CR process, and anytime anything happens to him, he asks for a session with me. One time, he'd fallen off a earthmover and injured his leg and hip. When the doctor prescribed pain pills and set up a physical therapy program, my son checked first with me. We found that he had been offered a promotion at work and had hurt himself to avoid taking the position. At least, that was what his mind was projecting. Once we cleared the fear of taking more responsibility, the pain disappeared and his injuries quickly healed up.

Case #29. At a lecture, a man describes himself as successful at everything he does. He has the big home, several cars, a plane, a yacht, and all the right memberships in all the socially and politically correct organizations. However, he recently realized that all his success is in the material world, that he is a workaholic, and that all his success and validation have come from his ability to create wealth.

After attending my first lecture, he knows there is something missing in his life. When he discusses the direction of their marriage with his wife, she tells him that she is well satisfied with their lavish lifestyle and does not share his curiosity about the spiritual aspect of life.

In session, we discover that his motivation to acquire material things and give his family everything they want is to get validation and self-worth. He realizes that his parents never gave him the unconditional love he craved. They gave him material things, calling that love, and he is doing the same thing. We clear the program and reinstal the self-love and self-validation program. However, when he tries to discuss his new focus with his wife, she wants nothing to do with his new direction, nor is she going to participate in it. As a result, they divorce. He decides to drop the superficial social life style and simply enjoy the money he has. He tells his wife he is dropping out, and if she wants to continue the old way, she can pay for it herself. He changes his life completely and finds genuine happiness.

Case #30. A women volunteers at one of my lectures. We go through the basics of clearing and find that she has a severe thyroid deficiency, about which she is concerned because she is pregnant. Six months ago, her doctor told her that her thyroid test showed very low, so he prescribed thyroid supplement. However, she was under extreme stress at the time of the doctor visit, and that's why her thyroid function was down. The doctor was an authority figure, so her mind accepted his diagnosis.

We forgive the doctor for making the statement, and reprogram the mind's belief. After about fifteen minutes, her thyroid resumes normal operation and has continued to do so for many years.

Case #31. In lectures, I have demonstrated that most people do not love themselves nor will they allow others to do so. In this process, I ask the audience to repeat an affirmation in which we state: "I am entitled to live in peace, happiness, harmony, and joy."

Quite often people will leave out one of the words, as when one woman left out "harmony." We even repeated the affirmation, and she left it out again, while claiming to have said it. All 125 of the audience chimed in and said, "No you didn't."

After the third time, she included harmony in the affirmation, but when I told her I felt she needed to see me as a client, she refused. It is obvious she is in denial and that a denial-of-denial sub-personality is running her life.

Case #31. Another major find is the discovery of the denial and denial-of-denial sub-personalities. I have been working with a client for a few sessions and he seems to accept and hold the love program, yet I notice in his relationship with his family that he doesn't seem to follow through in how he communicates with them.

In the next session, I check for denial-of-denial in the love program. It appears that he loves himself and will receive love from others, but when we check denial sub-personalities, they indicate he is in denial, that he does not love himself nor will he accept love from others.

When we release the denial sub-personalities and begin tracing back for the core issues, we find tremendous anger and suppressed resentment at his mother which in turn has created a resentment toward all women. This, too, is in denial. As we process through this, it opens many other doors to other suppressed denial programs and sub-personalities.

Case #32. Love and validation are the most important issues in a child's life. In my case, it was the base cause of all my problems. My parents did not know how to express love or give validation so it was the core issue in most of my dysfunctional behavior.

With one client, we found that his parents provided all the things that a child would want, private prep school education, and all the trappings to go with it. However, all they provided was material objects; there was no love, validation, or acceptance. The child tried to satisfy his parents for providing all the proper things in his life, but could never perform up to their standards. No matter how well he did, they always wanted more or better. Most of time, he received invalidation rather than acceptance.

Being a survivor, he went into business for himself and succeeded, but again received no support for his success. Finally, he even rejected his own self, and manifested a life-threatening disease to win his family's acceptance. He was willing to destroy himself for acceptance.

This shows how far the mind will go to get love and acceptance. He was not aware that his disease was caused by his mind setting him up. The doctors gave him a "no way out" diagnosis. He turned to alternative processes and nutritional programs, but they did not work either. Finally, he was referred to me by a friend who'd had positive results from working with me.

In four sessions, we create a miracle. We clear the dysfunction with reprogramming and let go of his anger and resentment, coming to peace with his parents. Most of the programs are in denial so he is not even aware of them. Once we let go of all the denial, and he can love and forgive his parents, and the miracle of healing happens naturally.

Case #33. A couple is trying to sell their house but they are not sure where they want to move to, so they have not made any plans for the future. The house is not over-priced or in disrepair, but it just does not sell. The couple is really frustrated because they cannot move forward. They come to me assuming that there must be a curse or hex on them or the house, but we find nothing that is stopping them. However, we do find a tremendous fear of not having an anchor or security. The house is security that they cannot let go of. Although they have consciously decided to sell the house, their fear of not having security is blocking the sale. It is hard for them to let go of the security.

For the next 30 days, they write out long hand 21 times a day, "It is safe to sell the house. Security is an internal personal quality, not an outer physical situation."

As children, neither had had a solid home, and felt that if they let go of the house, they would be homeless. The mind is not rational, nor does it see how it acts out its fear. This is actually a double-bind. Consciously they wanted to sell the house, but they were subconsciously blocking the sale. This is one of the main reasons we have to locate and release all our childhood fears and emotional trauma. I had worked with them on other issues, yet this one escaped our notice until the house was on the market. Denial is so insidious that it's almost impossible to see its covert operation.

Case #34. At a lecture, a woman asks me what causes hypoglycemia. I explain, "Almost all sugar-based problems are caused by lack of love, and sugar, especially chocolate, which responds in the body like feeling loved."

"I was helping a friend put out a newsletter, and we planned to stick the address labels and take the newsletters to the post office by three. I was supposed to be at my friend's house at noon but I didn't show up until two. My friend was angry at me for not showing up on time, and had almost finished the job on her own."

"What was your reaction to your friend's anger?"

"I felt unappreciated for the work I'd already done, and headed directly to the candy shop. I bought a pound of jelly beans and ate them all in less than an hour. As a result, my hypoglycemic condition kicked in and I had a low blood-sugar blackout. At the hospital emergency room, they gave me an insulin shot."

I ask her, "So, what do you think the lesson was in that incident?"

Typical of a person in denial, she says, "It was my friend's fault. She made me go to the candy store."

"Okay, I suggest a session to clear the programs that are causing the situation."

During the session, she disagrees with me about the cause and claims she has perfect parents, so they are not the cause. I agree that they are not the cause, but that it is her reaction to how they've treated her that's causing the problem. She disagrees with my interpretation, and I do not see her again. Unfortunately, this classic case of denial-of-denial occurred before I knew how to deal with it.

Case #35. My client has a controlling mother-in-law who can't help taking over every dinner party, whether it's at her house or the homes of her adult children. We go over the issue and it find that it is non-acceptance coming directly from childhood. My client's mother has passed on but had the same controlling qualities. She could not keep her comments or her need to control to herself.

The client recognizes her mother's controlling patterns and lets them go. We release all the "I am not all right" programs, rejection as a child, and the feeling of inadequacy, along with loving and forgiving her mother-in-law. We then work on reclaiming personal power and taking control of her life so she will not react to her mother-in-law. We release her fear of standing up for herself and speaking out about how she feels.

When she hosts the next Christmas dinner, she tells her mother-in-law, "I can handle the kitchen. Why don't you spend time with the family. Dinner will be ready in a couple hours."

The mother-in-law grumbles at first, but finally complies.

When my client asks for clarification, I explain, "The only reason your mother-in-law took control is that everyone let her. They were reacting from their childhood programs. Now that you've taken your power back and no longer have any feelings of inadequacy around your mother-in-law, she can't grind with you. You are stronger than she is, so she backs down. Controllers are only as strong as other people will allow them to be. They'll always defer to a person who is in their own power. They can't intimidate those who are in control of their life."

Case #36. It seemed that everything this client did was intended to reject self, and that his parents had deliberately set out to destroy his self-worth as he was growing up because nothing he did was right by them. They found fault with everything he did, no matter how well he did it. He did well in school in the lower grades, but they offered no support validation, so he just gave up and barely graduated.

As an adult, he received validation for the work he did which helped some. Even then, however, he would sabotage himself. I was surprised that he came to me for help, because the more ingrained the behavior, the longer it takes to clear it. It was hard for him to understand, however, that he has drawn people into his life that would validate his self-image.

Many clients come with some form of back pain along their spine. In his case, it is middle back pain, just below the shoulder blades. This almost always signals self-rejection, and usually it begins *in utero*.

He has been going to a chiropractor twice a week but the adjustments will not hold. However, as we work out the self-rejection, his back pain begins to lessen and eventually disappears. It takes many sessions to finally clear all the childhood programs and resultant patterns as an adult. I am surprised at his commitment; he persists until we've cleared them. Most people gave up when the going gets rough.

Case #37. In 1998, we discovered how powerful the Conscious Rational Decision Making Mind is. I was shifting my focus from the Subconscious Mind and Ego being the control factor, yet I had not encountered the true power in the mind. When I ran headlong into auto-pilot, I knew I had hit the jackpot.

I was working with an established client and we encountered some locked-in programs when I discovered that auto-pilot is in the Conscious Mind. It partitions off a segment of the Conscious Mind and sets up its own operating system with sub-personalities to drive it.

After discovering this, I decide we must erase this system so we can take its power back from it. Little do I know how powerful it is. We are removing some of the sub-personalities when the client starts browning out, so I decide to clear the whole thing at once with the help of my cadre of reprogrammers, Ego and Subconscious Mind, Holographic Mind, Higher Self, Holy Sprit and Presence of God.

We begin with our affirmations to clear the programs and ask them to uninstall the operating systems of auto-pilot and delete, erase and destroy all the operating programs, patterns and operating instructions in the auto pilot. I reason that if we can get them all before she passes out, we will have it cleared. All I'd have to do is get her back in her body and we'd be finished. However, I don't realize that we've crashed her entire operating system. (She'd been on auto-pilot control 85 percent of her life.)

I can't wake her, and it takes two hours for her mind to reconfigure the operating system, plus another hour to get the programs functioning in the proper manner.

Now, before destroying auto-pilot, I ask how much control clients have over their lives. I now chip away at auto-pilot until I can de-install the operating system with knocking them out of their body. In her case, the client was wondering why she had behavior patterns she didn't like yet they manifested anyway. She was running double-binds, fighting auto-pilot for control. Fighting sub-personalities was disconcerting and exhausting, but now she has her power back, she sleeps less and has more physical energy.

Case #38. At a lecture, a woman asks, "Is it possible that I set up my husband to beat me up? He denies hitting me, but I have the bruises to prove it. Our relationship is good and this only happens once in while. There doesn't seem to be any reason for it as far as I can see."

When we begin testing for the indication, we run into major denial. The husband is not consciously aware that he is beating his wife, even though he can see the bruises. We establish that he blacks out during the episodes.

I was actually seeing what happened but I had to get him to experience it himself to breakout of the denial and illusion. So I asked him, "Who appears or what happens before you black out?"

At this point I could not get any further. Conventional psychology would be stumped at this point because, due to denial-of-denial, he has no recall whatsoever. It simply did not exist in his reality.

We have to access the fear causing the denial, so using the acupuncture points with N/CR, we see that his mother abused him as a child, and that he would escape into his magical child to avoid the yelling and pain. He would actually escape this reality into another magical reality that he had created.

With this established in his mind, we can then recall the incident. When we go through the process of releasing his mother and forgiving her, we open the door to reconstructing the incident. I explain to him what has happened and what he did to escape. He describes it thus: "When my wife starts ragging on me, I don't see her anymore. All I see is my mother's image overlaid over my wife's. I become a child and go into a place of seclusion to escape her. At that point, I don't remember anything until I come back. When I do come back, I'm disoriented and it takes a while to regain my balance."

We work on her need to attack him verbally, and get over her need to control and manipulate him, so the whole behavior pattern for both of them is cleared. A few months later, the wife tells me there have been no more incidents since.

With conventional psychology, this would probably have ended in divorce, which neither one wanted. How many of these types of cases have the same root cause, but end up in divorce court or jail time, when they can so easily be resolved?

Case #39. Many clients have said, "I knew getting married was a mistake, but I did it for my parents."

Many people get married for all the wrong reasons. Most of time, we marry one of our parents with whom we have not completed our lessons. We then transfer our neediness from the parent to the other person, which creates a new mother/son or father/daughter relationship. This will work until one partner gets tired of being controlled or not being given the attention they want. In men, it will result in sexual maladjustment because you cannot have sex with your mother. In women, this does not seem to cause any problem.

Many people are caught in relationship addiction so they will say they are addicted to love which they never get. Usually they do not have a functional love program in the mind's computer so they keep chasing what they think is love, when it usually is sex which they interpret as love. I find very few people who are actually happy in their marriage. Most of them coexist because it's "the right thing to do." Society and religion place so many rules and pressures on people that very few even really know what true happiness is.

If both people are willing to work on it together, a couple can sometimes resolve their differences and create a good relationship. When I have been able to work with both partners, we can release all the childhood programs with the parents and put the marriage back together. However, if one person changes and the other wants to continue on the same path, irreconcilable differences will probably lead to divorce.

In Studs Turkels book *Working*, he interviewed 30,000 people and found that only 5 percent were actually happy to the point that they would not change anything in their life. 15 percent were relatively happy and had a few things they would change. Another 20 percent were trying to change their lives but felt frustrated in their effort. But a whopping 60 percent were not happy with their life, and felt locked in with no way out. *This is a pretty sad commentary on life.* And worse, this book was written in the seventies; things have gotten much worse since then.

Case #40. Many clients have faced a major battle due to their body being toxic and out of balance, both in electrolytes and homeostasis. Candida is primarily a breakdown in sugar metabolism, and is one of the most difficult dysfunctions to overcome because it also has an insidious emotional component.

Many of my clients with candida have victim tendencies and a hard time disciplining themselves.

In one case, the client has followed the candida diet rigorously, yet is making no headway. After about three years, she is so weak from the diet that she quits her job. Then her disability runs out. When we start working, her ability to withstand cold is gone to the point she keeps her apartment at 80 degrees. She is so careful with her diet that it seems almost obsessive.

After five sessions, she is functional in her life. The base cause is childhood rejection. She had been an only child and a "mistake," since her parents did not want any children. However, they feel sorry for her and enable her candida by giving her money when the disability runs out.

Her base feeling is that nobody likes her and will dump her from a job at the first chance, which she proves right by setting herself up to get laid off. I am able break through the denial that she does not want to work because she would get fired. We clear the program and sub-personality, and her candida begins to clear up. Once she feels empowered to stand up for herself, she risks eating foods that in the past have caused her candida to flare up. She is surprised when this doesn't happen.

She knows we are making progress where no medical doctors have been able to find an answer, and after almost a year of weekly sessions, she starts sponsoring me and setting up lectures for me. However, after she recovers, her empowerment goes to the other extreme. Her anger at men comes up, something that often happens when a female client reclaims her power. Resentment surfaces from having been held down in the past, and they become aggressive and arrogant. Fortunately, most clients recognize their misplaced anger and recover.

Case #41. I meet many people who run into major blocks while working out, almost all of them caused by emotional limitations. When we release the emotional causes from the body, miracles happen.

A weight lifter is upset that he has paid his entry fee into a weight lifting contest but cannot lift more than 175lbs, when the minimum to enter the preliminary level is 300lbs. He is at a loss as to why he is suddenly so weak.

By asking a few pointed questions, I see the base cause, so I offer him a free session. He had a fight with his girlfriend and she left him for another man. His interpretation was that the other man was more desirable and had a better-looking body.

First, we release all the anger at his mother, and then at the girlfriend. We recover from his failed relationship, and from not being acceptable because he does not physically match up to the other man. We recover his self-esteem and clear the need to have someone else validate him. Two days later, he lifts 325lbs. He remarks that he has no idea what we did, but that it worked.

Case #42. At a lecture, a woman asks me, "Do you believe in hereditary diseases?"

As we saw earlier, I do not accept the concept of the hereditary passing on of disease. Both her husband and her son died recently of a heart condition they believed was hereditary. When we check her with kineisology, her Body/Mind confirms that they both died from a belief. If they had not held that belief, they would be alive today. I have proven over and over that beliefs can kill.

Case #43. A client tells me she is affected by environmental illnesses. We trace her belief back to her arrival from Europe at Ellis Island. It was an old ship and the odors of bunker fuel permeated the decks of the ship. The day before the ship docked, she lost contact with her mother and didn't find her until they disembarked. Her allergies and her sensitivity were directly connected to the fear of losing her mother. Once we released the fear, the sensitivity immediately disappeared.

Case #44. A client capitulates to anything her husband wants. She puts up with his verbal abuse because that is the way she was treated as a child.

One of main blocks to awareness is giving power away to an authority figure, regardless of who it is. It could be a parent, a friend, an employer, or a marriage partner. Outside observers will puzzle over the person being treated badly or with no respect, but the codependent accepts the mistreatment because of fear of being rejected. This usually goes back to childhood where children felt they were not accepted. As a result, they rejected themselves as "not all right." To get the "alrightness" back and get validated, they look for a person who appears to need them.

I always warn clients with this complaint that they should ask their partner to participate in the process or they may have fireworks when they become aware, empowered and reclaim their personal power.

After five sessions, the client asks her husband for a divorce. In an attempt to save the relationship, he has a few sessions with me, but refuses to do any follow up. They divorce soon after.

Case #45. The other side of the coin are the counter-dependents who are actually more fragile than the codependents. It's hard for them to see their need to be in control all the time. Most are so in denial of their behavior that they justify all their reactions to a given stimuli. When confronted with an issue, they will go into either flight or fight. To give in is to lose their power. Quite often they will resort to verbal abuse to maintain control.

It is hard to get a counter-dependent to recognize that civilized behavior does not mean losing your power. I strive to work with the client's partner in hopes that if the codependent reclaims his or her power, the partner will see the light, but this seldom happens.

Although a few clients are able to change the course of their future to happiness, joy and unconditional love, most of these cases sadly end in divorce.

Case #46. Many people who maintain "I have been on the spiritual path for 20 years or more, and have my life together" will volunteer to work at N/CR lectures and workshops. However, I contend that spiritual work cannot begin until we have built the foundation. All but three people I have checked who claim to have been on the spiritual path for 15 years or more have accomplished little if any real growth on their path. The cause is clear.

One such woman, a 20-year veteran of spiritual work, volunteers to demonstrate with me at a lecture. As I go through my basic checks, we find that her polarity is switched and she's out of her body. She does not love herself nor can she receive love from others.

I check for the cause, and find that she had a controlling mother who rejected her before she was born and didn't want any more children. All her life, she felt rejected and abandoned by her mother. Her list of programs is endless, so I suggest that she see me for a session where we could release all this and get her on the track to reclaiming her personal power and empowering herself.

The first treatment appears to work but blows her out from her reality even further because we destroyed her fragile operating system. In in a second session, we build a new operating system which allows her get on with building the foundation to launch into her spiritual work.

This has happened to more people than I can count. Instead of starting on the bottom step, they jump up to step 12. With a crumbling foundation under them, they crash when we bring up the emotional dysfunction in their life that has been covered up in denial-of-denial sub-personalities. The illusion is that they were growing, but because it's not done thoroughly, the mind just runs with an illusion. They assume that they've done all the basic work, when in fact, none of the releasing has happened, other than cathartic release.

This unfortunate experience often happens because of misdirected teachers and pseudo-shamans. Quite often people, embark on a spiritual path with no guidance, and assume that they can acquire the tools without guidance. In my experience, true clearing requires an accomplished teacher who can direct one on the path. The "I can do it all myself" attitude simply does not work.

Case #47. A person at my health club had a tragic experience because of his daughter's relationship addiction. She had broken up with her boyfriend because he was verbally abusive. He would alternate between staying away from her and harassing her. The father got a court restraining order to keep him away, and he disappeared for about six months. She was living with her father for protection so he felt safe for her. The old boyfriend called up and wanted to see her one last time before he moved out of state. She agreed to meet him at a restaurant nearby to talk with him.

Her father wanted to go along for protection, but she declined, saying that it was a large, busy restaurant. Apparently, their discussion became an argument, and the boyfriend pulled a gun, killed her, and then himself. "Why?" asked the father.

When one person gets paranoid over another, the latter becomes the medicine. If the aggressor cannot have his medicine, then no one else can. They see no reason to live, and feel they can take the person with them in death. Until we recently stopped looking at crimes of passion as a criminal act, they were inexplicable.

Case #48. With many clients, I find that the mind seems to be our enemy. As we saw before, the problem is not our Ego at all, but the Middle Self and its auto-pilot programs. Our mind decides it will protect us from the ultimate enemy: rejection, abandonment, invalidation and fear of failure. In an effort to protect us, it sets up sub-personalities to keep us from situations that might cause us to face what it feels will be failure. We can use willpower to force the issue and punch through it, but unfortunately that creates an inner conflict that wears us out.

Clients often tell me that they know that what they are doing will work well, but for some reason, it's not successful. The base cause is always: "I'm not all right," and "I'm not acceptable."

Self-rejection and invalidation are the core issues. When we clear these programs, things begin to work out. I have studied people who succeed in their life pursuits, and they always come from a functional family. You may ask, "Why not me? I've tried hard to be successful."

It all comes back to karma and the lessons you have to clear up now. The sooner the better. Do it now!

Case #49. A psychotherapist who specializes in children's issues brings a young client whose parents are involved with a cult that practices Black Magic ritual abuse. The child has been subject to the cult's practices and has been the target of ritual abuse.

When the mother divorced the father and broke away from the cult, she took the child to a psychotherapist to deal with the fear laid in by the ritual abuse. After three fruitless sessions, the young boy would not talk at all. The therapist told the mother she could do nothing and suggested a session with me.

In the session, I suggest going into the records to discover the source of the child's resistance to the therapist. We find that the child was reacting to the therapist's Meta-Communication which was being influenced by a past life when the therapist had practiced ritual abuse. Amid much emotional release and tears, we cleared the past life record and locked it in the archives so there would be no Meta-Communication about this experience.

The next time the child saw the therapist, he opened up and would not stop talking. In two sessions, using some N/CR processing along with conventional therapy, he was cleared of all the ritual abuse. This case shows how Meta-Communication functions; neither person knew what they were reacting to but it stopped the therapy cold. Resolution was a win-win for both therapist and client.

Case #50. The issue of attraction to the same sex is one of the most controversial issues I've had to deal with in my practice.

Are gay people actually born with homosexual pattern in their life? My answer is no, and I have documented proof. I have worked with many women and men on the issue, none of whom actually came to me to deal with that issue. Most of the time, they just have the same issues that everyone else has.

The client's mother had been a US Army nurse who married in the Philippines during WWII. The daughter was born in the Philippines into a functional and financially stable family, from whom the child received much love and affection. After the war, the parents returned to the US and the mother's family did not accept the Filipino father at all. In this family group, the mother and her family rejected the child, and the father was the only person who gave the young girl any affection and love.

After about five years, the father couldn't handle the abuse and rejection, and returned to the Philippines. If she'd been older, the daughter might have gone with him, but she grew up feeling rejected and abandoned by her father. The mother wouldn't let her visit her father for fear she wouldn't come back. It was like ownership but no affection or love.

Assuming that all men would reject her, my client gravitated to same-sex relationships. I asked her, "Why did you come to see me when you hate men so violently?"

"I feel that you're here to help me through the problems in my life. You never tell me how to run my life because you always give choices. I feel that you are a historian giving me back my childhood and helping me release the hatred and misplaced anger I've held on to until now. I feel at peace in my life now that I understand the causes for my behavior. This doesn't mean I'll be attracted to men, but now I know I have choice. Thank you for giving me back my life."

Case #51. At one of my lectures, a man asked, "Do you really believe that AIDS is not a disease?"

I replied, "It's not AIDS that kills people but the other viruses and bacteria that the immune system is unable control because of the low T-cell and leukocyte blood count. In fact, the AIDS virus mutates so fast that it destroys the immune system and there is no way to control it."

"Okay, are you willing to work with my friend."

"Of course," I replied. "AIDS is not contagious."

For such an advanced case, the results were dramatic. After just a week, the client stopped needing blood transfusions and his T-cell count shot up at an unheard of rate. The couple went on a vacation they'd been planning for years, but had had to postpone indefinitely. The client died within two weeks of their return. The official cause was listed as AIDS but, on further pathological studies, no cause of death could actually be pinpointed. The friend (who had attended my lecture) was HIV positive and now wanted to ensure that it did not develop into AIDS.

We clear up the HIV status in two weeks, and he continues to have sessions with me for about a year. By the end of the year, he is questioning his same-sex attraction, and is now in a heterosexual relationship.

Case #52. A psychologist friend referred a lesbian who was having relationship problems with her partner. After a basic session, she wants to know why she took on the lesbian lifestyle. We unwind the core issues and the original cause: intense anger at her father and all of the men in her life. During the sessions, she releases her anger, and decides to opt out of the lesbian lifestyle. Her partner is furious and comes to see me.

The session with the partner is one of the most tumultuous sessions I've experienced. She begins by screaming at me, "You destroyed my relationship. I feel like committing suicide. Carolyn left me for man. She has penis envy and I can't provide satisfying sex for her."

After she gets that off her chest, I ask, "Well, what do you want to do about it?" Apparently, she just wanted to unload on me. Soon after, she calls to apologize and book a session. In several sessions, we release the anger and many of the issues around the rejection, and she reclaims her personal power which opens her up for more effective relationships.

Case #53. I was invited to present a lecture by a women who had attended a lecture with a friend from distant city. Unknown to me, of the 28 attendees, only three were heterosexual. In my ignorance, I answered questions without any withholds and the audience accepted my answers without much resistance.

At the end of the lecture, a women asked me if I would stay after the lecture and work on her. She'd been afraid to volunteer during the lecture because she could feel her anger rising. She warned me that she would probably begin screaming during the release. She was right; she did, at the top of her voice.

Afterwards, she told me she felt like a piece of spaghetti. In a further session, we clear mountains of rejection and anger against her father and men in general, which gave her a new life. She has no intention of relinquishing her lesbian lifestyle, but the clearings gives her a whole new life. Her "male rejection" issues are the same as for many women, yet her interpretation had guided her into a lesbian lifestyle.

Case #54. Two of my clients are cross-dressers. One keeps trying to start relationships with women even though he knows they will eventually reject him. The pattern is that he chooses a strong, controlling woman who wants a mother-son relationship. He then rebels because he tries to prove to himself that he's male when his inner self really wants to be a women, and he reacts as a man or woman depending on the situation, although he seems happier in the female persona. Either way, his intended female partner rejects him.

His background was typical of transsexual men, covered in Chapter 2, but he was terrified of the sex change option. Unfortunately, he stopped the sessions, so we didn't reach resolution.

Case #55. The client's life-stress was simply breaking his body down, and his adrenal function was so low that he should have been totally shut down by clinical depression, yet amazingly, due to the power of the mind, he was still somehow able to function, even though exhausted all the time. He was a survivor and was using pure will power to drive his life. Once we released all the childhood trauma and he reclaimed his personal power, he began to recover and is now able to function normally.

Case #56. Occasionally a sick client is getting a payoff from his or her illness, often related to control of others. Asthma is commonly the illness of choice to manipulate other people who then give their power to the controller. I have explained to many controllers what they're doing to get the payoff, yet most deny it.

In some cases, we may have cleared all the programs, beliefs, and sub-personalities from every level of the mind, yet if they retain the concept of payoff in the Conscious Rational Mind, it will rebuild the program, and the disease syndrome will return. I have cleared some clients of asthma for up to two weeks, yet it returns with more intensity than in the past.

Case #57. Fear of stepping forward or reaching out in life can result in pain or physical breakdown in our arms in legs. At an Expo, I met a women with a paralyzed arm who had no use of the fingers on her left hand. One morning, ten years ago, she woke up ten years ago with her hand in this position. After much physical therapy, she could move her arm, but nothing seemed to help her hand.

In the first session, we trace the original cause to her childhood, when her parents told her she would not succeed at anything. They invalidated everything she did. Ten years ago, she was going to start a new job in which she would have to use her hands, and to make sure she couldn't fail, her programming had kicked in to prevent her from taking the job.

Once we release the parental programming and the fear of failure, she is able to reclaim her personal power. We also reprogram her love program so she can love herself and allow herself to receive love. We release the fear of reaching out to new situations and new realities. Her arm loosens up, and her hand uncurls, right in the session, to give her full use of her fingers for the first time in ten years.

Case #58. A client lived only a few blocks from my office, and was a virtual prisoner in his house. He was afraid to go out due to what he described as "environmental illness" in that he was allergic to everything.

We begin with his pre-birth rejection by his mother—she didn't want any children. She verbally and physically abused him, and wore strong perfume all the time, so he connected rejection and abuse with strong perfume. With a shy victim-type personality, it was no surprise when he married a strong, controlling woman who verbally abuses him and controls his life. He was seeking a mother-son relationship so that he could continue to work out relationship lessons with his mother. She also wears strong perfume, which is the core issue.

The client used to work at a scientific laboratory that used strong-smelling chemicals—the catalyst. He developed reactions to the chemicals, and finally retired on disability. His allergy syndrome built on itself until, today, he is afraid to go anywhere.

We clear all the childhood programming with his mother. Then we tackle the beliefs and sub-personalities that are driving the concepts about environmental illness. Once clear, we take a field trip to a lecture to try out his newfound freedom.

As fate would have it, a women with strong perfume sits down right behind us, and he bolts for the door to get some fresh air. Outside, I manage to convince him that his environmental illness is a self-created illusion, and we go back in and enjoy the rest of the lecture. Over the next few sessions, we clear his remaining problems, finally releasing him to find happiness and joy for the first time in his life.

Case #59. A prospective client called from Florida, but since I live in California, meeting was a problem. As it happened, Ft. Lauderdale was hosting an upcoming Expo, so we arranged to meet there.

He had been diagnosed as a classic case of learning-disabled, coupled with ADD. His family had sent him to many therapists but to no avail. At their suggestion, he enrolled in a college that helped learning-disabled people, but after five years, he was still in his junior year. He was listless, and had difficulty getting out bed each morning and just making it through the day.

As usual, his problems all stemmed from childhood during which he collected the usual rejection programs in addition to his father continually putting him down. He did poorly in school, and was unable to fit into the social scene. When his school labeled him learning-disabled, he bought it hook, line and sinker.

In the first session, we clear the ADD label and learning-disabled belief, along with all the traditional programs. Immediately, he begins to find school easy. He is amazed that we could release pain in his body and change his programming and belief by just holding acupuncture points on the body and saying an affirmation. Over two more sessions, he reclaims his personal power and takes responsibility back, and perks up in every area of his life. He jumps out of bed, eager to tackle each day, and wants to be up and around. He tells me, "I've never felt like this before. Now I have this drive to succeed and get going in my life."

Case #60. In the mid-80s, a women came to my lecture dressed like a construction worker. She wore Levis, heavy work boots and a flannel shirt. She said, "I fit into one of the categories you talked about, and I want to find out why."

For the last 15 years, she'd installed new electric lines for the power company, and was the only woman she knew of in construction.

She was the youngest of three girls. Her parents had wanted a boy but were unwilling to have a fourth child. She'd been a tomboy all her life, playing sports and generally spending most of her time with men, stopping at bars with her crew for an after-work drink. She had no boyfriends or intimate relationships, even though men would show interest in her. She'd never had lesbian tendencies, nor did she want any part of that lifestyle. Interestingly, she didn't feel rejected by her parents, or that they'd treated her like a boy. She just took on that lifestyle herself to prove to her father that she could meet his demands on her.

We release the programs about needing to please her parents, and she reclaims her personal power so she can live her life for herself. She comes to her second session wearing a dress, and I ask, "What happened?"

She replied, "The need for the challenge isn't there anymore. I don't feel I have to prove anything to my parents. I just want a lifestyle where I can live a normal life, so I applied for a transfer to the dispatch department with an inside/outside combination position."

This client is typical of people who just flow with the river, not really directing or controlling their lives, but who do not experience happiness and joy. Once she got in touch with, and understood her choices, she changed path to one more in line with what she desired. Her new lifestyle brought her peace, harmony, happiness, and joy. She began a good relationship with a new male friend, with whom she could work on the love aspect. She also began to make women friends.

Case #61. One of the questions that puzzles many people is, "I want to clear up patterns in my life, so why can't I accomplish what I set out to do?"

One client had cleared all the blocks to accomplishing her goals, yet in the next session, we found that she was self-sabotaging. The culprit is a program buried in her Conscious Rational Mind, hidden in denial. Its thinking is that if she does not keep her commitments, nobody could hold her responsible, so she could never fail. She would get migraine headaches to stop her from achieving her goals, but then she'd feel guilty for not keeping to her commitment, and she'd berate herself for not following through. She justified the pattern by saying that she needed compassion, but that others were critical of her, and withheld it.

Breaking this pattern takes several sessions, because between sessions, she recreates the programs and beliefs for the mileage she derives from them. When she finally realizes that her soap opera drama is costing her jobs and friends, she decides to reclaim her personal power. Her life rapidly turns around.

Case #62. During childhood, this client lost his father to serious illness, and his mother seriously neglected him. He came to me claiming that outside forces were plaguing him. I had my doubts but went along with the possibility.

We begin on the premise that outside forces are affecting his health, and over a few sessions, we clear all the outside effects being caused by other people. In his own mind, he had created blaming belief patterns that spawned many "denial of denial" blamer sub-personalities connected with a number of denial and "refusal to take responsibility" sub-personalities.

All told, we clear over 45 sub-personalities, but then his entire operating system crashes. He feels drugged, sick and congested, and unable to function. A later session uncovers a whole other set of the same programs and patterns. The problem was that with "denial of denial," a person cannot access the programs or patterns, so they seem real because, as far the client is concerned, the feelings are real. When we access the records, we find that some are old, but others are new, created to justify the aberrant behavior and feelings. So we keep chipping away at the programs, and at some point, we will clear them all. This process continues until the client either sees the truth or gets fed up with the way he feels.

Case #63. Similar cases arise when clients live in a dream world of fantasy. One client came to me quite disoriented, a condition psychologists call bipolar or manic depression. As usual, I looked for the original cause of his dysfunctional behavior.

The original cause was that when the client was very young, his father died. His mother never remarried and retreated into a dysfunctional state so she didn't have to take responsibility. As a teenager, therefore, he ended up taking care of her. An aunt helped out but essentially, he had no adult model to follow and felt massive rejection. As a survival mechanism, his mind suppressed the programs under layers of denial. (Of course, the rejection lesson will recur later in life.)

We find the base cause is denial of reality. He doesn't want to accept the lesson or what was happening to him. We find the core issue is not wanting to accept responsibility, plus denial-of-denial of responsibility sub-personalities, plus 30 denial-of-denial blamer sub-personalities. He can't even recognize his trait of walking into situations and setting himself up, because in his mind, everybody else is causing his problems.

When we start to remove all the blocks and erase the denial sub-personalities, he almost passes out. At the end of the first session, he is exhausted. In future sessions, we keep finding the same programs, but when we find the catalyst, he makes a major breakthrough and is finally able to get his life back on track.

Case #64. In my seminars, I always assert that any allergy is a belief that has no program driving it. Instead, it is driven by a sub-personality that is activated by the catalyst, something we can clear up in 15 – 30 minutes.

The client came to me after falling down in tall grass while running her dog, and within hours, suffering an allergic reaction. Her face swelled up and she got a red rash, with spots all over her body. However, her doctor couldn't find any actual allergy.

In session, we find the original cause was, as a child, being frequently beaten up in tall grass by her older brother. He was angry that she'd been born and was "stealing" his parents' attention away from him. Beating her up was his means of expressing his anger.

The core issue was created many years later when she got into knock-down fight with her ex-husband, also in tall grass. Tall grass became the catalyst, so every time she falls down in tall grass, her irrational belief says she's going to get beaten up. The allergy simply delivers the message that there's a lesson that has to dealt with, but she isn't able to hear it.

When we clear the belief, sub-personality, core issue and base cause, within 15 minutes, the swelling and rash disappear right before our eyes. Since the catalyst is now permanently erased, there is nothing to activate the issue, so the grass allergy will not recur. All it took was an appropriately-worded affirmation.

Case #65. At one of my lectures, a woman asked, "Your theory sounds great and I'd like to believe it, but I had back surgery and four ruptured disks removed. I can't deal with the pain any longer. It's so bad that I'm contemplating suicide."

I told her, "Please don't put the responsibility for your life on me because I'm only a programmer, not a healer. I don't heal anyone, but I can show you how to heal yourself. *You* have to rewrite the scripts and install the programs I provide you with."

In her first session, I learn that her parents were career Air force officers and didn't want any children, but if they did have one, they wanted a boy. She was an only child and saw very little of them, so she installed the self-rejection programming: "They don't want me; I'm not accepted."

Her back problems stemmed from her spine contracting from the trauma that was locked in by the programming. When the pressure of the muscle contraction became too intense, the disks ruptured. Doctors tried to fuse them, but it didn't work, so two years later, they surgically removed the disks and tied four of the vertebrae together with stainless steel wire. This didn't work either, so it's obvious to me that she was still not getting the message.

She decides to go for it, commits to healing herself, and the results are amazing. In the first session, we release the rejection, and the pain disappears. In the second, we discover and release some traumatic past lives with the same parents. But what we didn't know was that a miracle had already happened.

The client sets up an auto accident and has to have back X-rays. The doctor assumes he's mixed up two patient's X-rays, but when it's eventually proved that these *are* her X-rays, he is completely baffled because they show that the stainless steel wire has disappeared, all four disks are present, and the vertebrae are in perfect condition. The four discs that had been removed surgically are back in their original locations and perfectly healthy!

Some follow-up work clears the balance of the trauma, and in the last ten years, the client has had no back problems. Her body was talking very loudly, screaming even, but she was just not getting the lesson. The fact that her health turned around in just a feww days proves the power of the mind.

Case #66. One of the most phenomenal cases I have had involves a client I met at a lecture I did in Las Vegas. He is an extraordinary example of someone who succeeded against incredible odds.

Born with cerebral palsy, he couldn't speak until he was six. He was confined to a wheelchair and unable to move himself until he was eight. He started school late due to his disabilities, yet he graduated from high school in the normal time. He had a college degree, a B.Sc. in mechanical engineering, built race cars, and had won many races. He started his own business and was an inventor, patenting and building some of his own inventions. When we met, he still had some spastic body movements and slurred speech, one would assume from a stroke, say, but was able to live an almost normal life.

Very few people with cerebral palsy live beyond age 35 and can seldom take care of themselves or perform in a job above minimal responsibility. At 62, he had outlived anyone with cerebral palsy in past history.

He had the usual quotient of human emotional programming, plus tremendous anger at people who treat him as a disabled person who cannot do anything for himself. In his business dealings, people took advantage of him because they felt he could not defend himself. But he proved them wrong time and again, and succeeded beyond any expectations.

When I started working with him in 1996, he is beset by people trying to sabotage one of his inventions, so we change the negative programming causing the problems. We are still "work-in-progress" today, but I know nothing will stop him. His life path proves that nothing can stop you if you have the courage, commitment and the discipline to move through your limitations. He has never considered himself victim. He sees life as a challenge that one can overcome with commitment and consistent work.

Cerebral palsy is a Karmic genetic situation filed in the pre-birth flight plan. The Soul knows it can take this lesson on and overcome the effects of the so-called birth "defect." Here is a man who on his own was able to work through the disabling effect of cerebral palsy and succeed at making a life for himself with very little help. He is an excellent example of a person whose mind tells him he can't do what he's attempting, yet he does it anyway. How many of us could even begin to overcome such a challenging genetic life controlling "defect"?

Case #67. We were participating in a health show in February 2001 and hoped to see a friend who had helped me set up seminars and workshops for many years. When he came up to our booth, his condition appalled Susie and I. I assumed he would be participating at the show himself, but he was in no condition to do so. He was a well-known healer and reflexologist whom I had known for over 15 years but had not seem him for over a year. Therefore, I was shocked to see him so badly crippled that he had to use a walker. He could not talk clearly and was shaking with Parkinson's Disease. "What happened to you?" I asked him.

"I don't know," he told me. "No one seems to be able to help me. I've been to many practitioners I know who tried to work with me, but to no avail."

"I suggest you make an appointment with me and so we can clear all of the dysfunctional programs and heal your afflictions," I advised.

He did so and, when I worked with him, tracking the programs and clearing the files was quick and easy because we had done so much work together in the past. In one session, we healed the Parkinson's Disease and cleared his speech problem. He left the session without the walker and taking very clearly. Two days later, his lady friend called to say, "You have given Jim back to me. It's amazing what you have done with him."

Six months later, none of the afflictions have returned. All neuro-motor diseases are easy to clear once you find the base cause and clear the programming. The "Catch 22' is that the person has let go of the need for the illness. He was not getting any mileage out of his affliction, so it was easy to reprogram and release.

Case #68. I work with many people who cannot seem to get their life in gear, so they procrastinate all the time until a major crisis wakes them up. This happened to one client who was forced to take action in his life. When he was able to handle the situation, he found that it was so easy when he took responsibility that he decided to go forward on all his unfinished languishing projects. I saw him less than a month later, and he had total control over his life; auto-pilot was gone and he had no control sub-personalities.

I thought this was a miracle; the month before, he'd been loaded with sub-personalities that caused avoidance, disorientation and procrastination. And now they were all gone. Sowing the seeds over the last year had worked. Once he reclaimed his personal power, he was on track. The last time I saw him, he commented, "When you are on the other side of the fence, you can see all the denial and illusion other people are in, but they will not listen to you when you observe it in them."

I asked him, "Does that phrase sound familiar from our sessions?"

He grinned and said, "Now I'm in your shoes, I can see why I did not want to admit where I was. It sure is a lot more comfortable to be where I am now."

Case #69. One of the more amazing experiences I have had came up with a client who was slowly dying and we could not seem to stop her life simply slipping away. Eventually, we found that she had regressed into a past life where she'd had a condition similar to Alzheimer's. It was as if she was living in a parallel lifetime even though she seemed to be cognizant of things around her, yet other times, she would slip away into this other lifetime. The family had significant funds so it was not a matter of money. Our work revealed that she felt that she no longer had any opportunities in life. We would heal one condition and she would pull up another affliction until she became unable to move on her own.

Over a six-month period, she progressed from simple problems to life-threatening conditions, where she could not eat much at all. When I told her what she needed to do to halt the progression she was creating, I noticed myself getting to a point where I almost passed out. When I told the client's daughter what was happening, she astounded me by saying, "You actually did. You passed out for four minutes. It was like you just faded out and stopped talking for no reason."

Checking with Kinesiology, I discovered that her mind had knocked me right out of my body. It was intent on killing her and did not want me interfering. Nothing I could do could turn that intent around, even though the client was aware of what was happening. She finally died in her sleep about two weeks later.

The power of the human mind sometimes amazes me. Not only did it destroy her, but it also stopped me from helping her.

Case #70. During 2001, I began to find that many clients who have had a life-threatening illness feel that the battle of life is futile. To a few of them, this is a startling and shocking revelation, but most do not even recognize that this is happening to them. This attitude is activating what I call the Instinctual Mind's files, and few people know about this mind or what it can do to them. When these files are opened, they begin to create "I want to die" programs and "fear of dying" programs. In extreme cases, clients can have as many as 150 files open. The root cause of Alzheimer's is the battle between the "I want to die" and "I'm afraid to die" programs. When the programs are active for a long time, they create an Alzheimer's program that will advance slowly until short-term memory starts to be affected. Clearing and erasing these programs clears suicidal feelings and restores short-term memory.

In one of the most advanced cases, the client had written two books but could not seem to get them out to the market. We cleared her fear of failure around the books and assumed that everything would fall into place. However, the following month, the Instinctual Mind's file was open again with more "I want to die" programs. Then we found so many programs in denial-of-denial about her self-worth that had not been cleared that she was setting up a program to escape from life rather than confront potential failure. We finally broke through when we discovered a string of past lives paralleling her current challenge where she had backed out rather than confront the fear of success or failure.

A lesson you avoid in past lives will be forwarded to the current life until you get the lesson. Each time, the lesson is more intense until you recognize it. Here, the client blamed her failure on people who would not accept her work and others who dropped the ball when she needed help. They were unknowingly just cooperating with her program in order to force her to recognize the lesson. When she contacted these same people again, everything went according to clockwork and fell into place and on time. This is an example of something I tell many clients: this is an interactive universe and we all work in each other's lessons whether we want to or not.

Case #71. Our fear seems to surface when we least expect it. With the down-sizing of companies, many of my clients are in fear of being downsized out of a job. I had two recent cases involving down-sizing, both very different.

One client knew that he was going to get fired, so he retrained in another sector of the same field and became a consultant making more money than he had before.

Another very inventive client made herself indispensable. She performed all the backup work for her supervisor, who then had more free time to do the things she wanted to do but which were not really part of her job. When downsizing cut the department from 45 people down to 5, my client had no problem since she had been working with me to build her self-confidence and self-worth, and reclaim her personal power. She was able to weather the storm since she could handle the workload increase but her supervisor could not because she hadn't been keeping current with the workload since my client had taken so much of it on. Both of them had an increased workload, and my client refused to carry her supervisor's extra load as she had in the past. The supervisor is now trying to find a way to leave the company. Even though my client knew she might get laid off, she was able to handle the stress. She did activate a few programs around it but we were able clear them easily.

It is clear to me that the reason some people succeed is that they do not see themselves as losers and they evaluate what they can do to succeed. The most important qualities are self-esteem, self-worth and self-confidence, and that you know that you are entitled to abundance in your life. You can do anything you want to, if you believe that it is possible. Victims do not hold that belief.

Future revisions of this book will share more research and case histories. I have maintained contact with many of my clients over the years and they have all said that N/CR changed their life path for the better.

Chapter 15

The Practice of Neuro/ Cellular Repatterning

A Self Healing Process?

We would like to think we can heal ourselves, but after twenty years in the healing field, I know very few who have successfully managed to sidestep the mind's games. Many clients who claim to have cleared these issues themselves have attended a workshop where they learn some self-healing techniques and bingo, they think they can heal themselves. But when we actually access the issues, we find that at a conscious level, they believe they cleared them, but at the reality level, Subconscious Mind disagrees.

Few people listen to their body, or their mind, for that matter. If they did, we would not have so many deranged, dysfunctional, or sick people in our world. If people were aware of what their behavior causes, we would not have so many abused children, crimes and wars.

How about those who have studied alternative healing, are on a path to transformation, and are committed to working out their issues? I have found that more than 50 percent are in denial of many of the issues blocking their progress. What of the many teachers, shamans and therapists who claim to help people out of their past and create a new path to transformation?

All I ask for is documented, pragmatic verification that the process actually works in the longterm. How many people have had life-threatening diseases permanently eliminated from their life? How many people with physical disabilities have been healed so they never have pain again? Did the process help clients to find a long-lasting relationship with a partner? Were clients able to overcome obstacles that blocked financial success? Were they able to overcome fear and anger programs that were causing depression or chronic fatigue?

In the last 20 years, only two practitioners have been willing to give me names of clients I could talk to and verify that they were helped over the long haul. In developing N/CR, I was unable to find a process that would permanently clear my dysfunction. I spent a lot of money on seminars, workshops and therapists who assured me that they could clear my pain. Where does this leave us in our search for the truth in healing?

The human mind in denial is complex and intricate. The programs and sub-personalities deceive us so that they can protect us. Their irrational interpretation makes no sense when looked at logically. After ten years research, I discovered how the mind processes information: it functions as a computer. But how can lay people use this information to heal themselves?

Some clients have been able to make progress once I worked with them to clear the basic programs. Some did not need much help from me because they had been working on themselves for many years and were able to make considerable progress. How did they do it? Willingness to be totally open to change; refusal to blame anyone or anything for the problems that faced them; taking total responsibility for every situation in their life; determination; commitment to their purpose; consistent concentrated effort to follow through with their journey to enlightenment.

Discipline and discernment are the most important qualities in the quest. Denial and illusion will try to trip you up at every turn. Auto-pilot will stop you dead in your tracks by creating the illusion of success.

How much control we have over our lives determines our ability to use self-healing techniques and reclaim our personal power from the Middle Self's sub-personalities that operate auto-pilot. Discernment reveals the many diversions on the path and helps us avoid grasping at anything that looks like it may provide direction. The path is littered with deceivers who genuinely believe that they're providing a service but are so deep in illusion and denial themselves they cannot even see the truth. This is not a judgment; it's an observation based on attending many seminars and workshops, and being a client with many therapists. The key word is discernment: evaluate what the therapist presents and ask many questions. If he or she is defensive, noncommittal or evades your questions, then steer clear. Use your discernment to avoid seeing so-called healers as authority figures because, as such, you may want to believe them. Be skeptical until the proof is before you.

So, can we heal ourselves? Maybe. Often you can get to simple issues that are causing localized pain, but to get to deeply-embedded or locked-in programs that are in denial takes a skilled practitioner. To be able to work on yourself, you must uncover the causes of dysfunction that you want to heal, correct or release. If you are clear on what the issues are, you might be able to access the information with practice. Begin with active meditation that puts you in contact with the Akashic Record.

To use Kinesiology, you must be clear of Middle Self's influence. It always wants to be right and control the process. It will block you from using any technique it cannot control (see below for a clearing process).

Pattern Release Process

This section indicates how to access and release beliefs, programs and sub-personalities:

Symptom: Mental, emotional or physical pain, depression, illness, etc. (obvious or assumed cause)

Record: Base cause, actual interpretation of situation, Subconscious Mind's recording of reaction, activity
or situation

Program: Core issue, Subconscious Mind's or Middle Self's
sub-personality instructions recorded in computer
(how I will handle situation next time).

Pattern: Habitual reaction, the illusion of how I have
handled the situation in the past whenever the
stimulus arose (addiction, control, justification,
denial, authority, distortion, dishonesty, delusion.)

Those who can access this information can work with N/CR
themselves, but few people are clear enough to do so. Sometimes,
the programs are so strong that they're right on the surface so
anyone can recognize them and release them, but most of the
time, they're deeply-hidden or in denial, and the deeper they are,
the harder it is to locate and access them. Even some clairvoyants
and clairaudients cannot read their own book.

Yes, I healed many of my blocks myself, but I could not get
to the deeply-buried issues. Ironically, they came up when I was
working with my clients and had to deal with them in a session.
By putting myself in the affirmation with the client, I was able to
release many of my own programs.

You may be able release or relieve a symptom yourself, and
achieve remission or release of pain, but this will not cause healing to take place. You are simply manipulating the energy tied up
in the neurological pathway, meridian, muscle, organ or tissue. If
you do not release the base cause and the core issue, the instructions will eventually cause the pattern to reassert itself when a
crisis issue arises in your life.

The Conscious Mind can set up a belief and the soul can understand the process, but if the Subconscious Mind does not release the record from the files and lock up the operating
instructions in the archives, the instructions will cause the computer to restore the program. It will continue to do so until the
pattern/program/record is recognized, filed and released with love

and forgiveness. Then, the original cell imprint can begin operating again, healing all the dysfunctional parts of the cell. The immune system can then regenerate, which allows the T-cells and leukocytes to resume their work. To activate the body's healing ability, the body must be able to access the original blueprint. When the programs are lifted from the cell memory, the body/mind will be able to heal the disease and/or emotional dysfunction.

After twenty years practice with N/CR, I can access almost anything and rewrite the program, thus healing it myself, but with programs and sub-personalities in denial of denial, I still need a practitioner to help me. However, if I cannot locate the cause, I do not get caught up in pride. My desire is to be as clear as quickly as possible, so I am not going to get trapped in the need to be in control or to manipulate the situation so I can look good. I have no need to have someone validate me for how effective I am at healing myself or my clients. Being a know-it-all, being in control, having to be an authority figure, arrogance and resistance do not get us anywhere. I often find these qualities in self-proclaimed "enlightened" people, yet they are unaware of these traits because they are held in denial. True seekers, on the other hand, shine out in their clarity.

The next section provides a format for setting up a session and the use of affirmations. The basis of all this work is to rewrite the software in the mind and redirect the manner in which the mind processes information.

The Neuro/Cellular Repatterning Session

Please note that this brief description does not equip anyone to perform a full treatment session. Neuro-kinesiology is described in separate booklet for those who want to study N/CR process in depth. A manual for N/CR is also available for those who plan to take the training. Cost is $95, which will be credited and applied to the cost for a level one workshop.

The basic processes use neuro-kinesiology (muscle testing) and do not require the practitioner to be clairvoyant, but it helps. Later steps do require clairvoyant or clairaudient ability.

The electrical polarity of the client's body must be balanced before we can begin a session. We are an electromagnetic mechanism, and must have our electrical polarity balanced in order to operate effectively. If it is reversed, we cannot get accurate answers. Most people's polarity is out of synch due to the stress and fear prevalent in today's world.

The purpose of N/CR is to remove defective software from the mind by deleting, erasing and destroying it. Once done, we install a new program or reinstate the original program that was blocked out and written over. This is done using an affirmation. The therapist cannot install programs on behalf of clients; clients must install the program themselves by repeating the affirmation after the therapist. This installs the program in the computer. The therapist must be observant and listen carefully when a client is repeating the affirmation so that every word is in the right sequence.

A client who skips a word or phrase indicates resistance, a heavy control program, or a sub-personality blocking the issue. The affirmations are specifically worded so as to release an old program or install a new one. Every word the mind takes in can have an effect on you.

To ask questions accurately, put one hand on the client's forearm and the other hand over the client's solar plexus (third chakra). This accesses the Subconscious Mind rather than the Middle Self.

The Use Of Neuro Kinesiology (Muscle Testing)

Basic Neuro Kinesiology checks

Two important tools of N/CR are the use of affirmations and Kinesiology. These two modalities give us the means to locate the files in the body/mind.

My original training in Kinesiology was with Dr. John Diamond, the originator of Behavioral Kinesiology (BK). His unique methods reveal what the inner mind is holding. This is how he described BK at the time. "I did not understand in the beginning why, when using Kinesiology, putting my hand over my abdomen gave an answer that always seemed to be more accurate than arm-testing alone."

In my work, I have found this to be true 100 percent of the time, but I narrowed the location down to the solar plexus. I no longer check with the arm only (unless I am demonstrating how the two minds differ in their answers). Why do people who work with muscle testing use a process that is only marginally effective? Because they do not know that there is a more effective way. Diamond clearly knew that we received better answers in 1978. We have proven, without a doubt, that when you do not put your hand on the Solar Plexus when you test, you do not get accurate answers. You will find that you get totally different answers when you use the arm only.

When you find the client's arm is like an iron bar and will not go down with any question or pressure, there is something controlling the client's neurological system. This could turn out to be a contest of wills but, more often, it is the work of controlling sub-personalities or entity/being possession. You will have to clear the entities before you can begin any work.

There are many descriptions of Kinesiology. Everybody seems to put their own prefix on it to describe their individual process. We use "neuro" because we are asking the body to tap into the programs in the mind. It does this through the muscles' response through the neurological system. In actuality, all muscle testing works in this manner no matter what prefix you use. The mind is telling you what its response is through a neuro-synapse reaction. All muscle response is controlled by the mind. When you ask the question, it accesses the computer's database and reveals the answers. If you ask it to check a product to see if the client needs a particular nutrient, the mind will check the body and report back the answers. There are only three ways it can communicate: through intuitive projection, neuro-synapses or neuro-peptides.

I developed this process over the last 15 years. I found that I could pick up the answers without any outside means but many people did not believe what I was telling them so I decided I needed to develop a system to validate more definitively what I was describing. Neuro-Kinesiology is the result. I used my Behavioral Kinesiology training to develop my new method and we found a new avenue to help people answer questions without having to use their intuitive or clairvoyant abilities. We found that if we directed the mind to ask the question of the right source, then we could access anything, including the Akashic Record.

Clarity is of the utmost importance when using muscle testing, and there are many ways to use it. First and foremost, however, the practitioner must be clear (see next chapter).

You can use your mind's awesome abilities to talk to your own body or to God with the Kinesiology process just as easily as with any other technique. You can use any set of muscles that will give you an "up and down" action or an "open/closed" indication. Using fingers, you can hold your thumb and middle finger together and try to pull them apart. Using an arm or a leg, you ask the person to resist your pushing or pulling.

If a sub-personality is in control, you can tap on the thymus gland to regress or progress, or take the client's power down so you can test them. You say verbally, "Reduce available power to 30 percent," while tapping the thymus gland. (The thymus gland is located behind the collarbone just below the V-shaped bone below the neck.) Tap on the thymus gland and say to yourself, "Go back to three o'clock this morning." If that does not work, tap again and say, "Reduce the power down to 30 percent." This should work in a battle with Middle Self. (Remember to return the client to present time and full power before you finish. If you don't, it could cause problems.)

If you are unable to get accurate answers with Kinesiology, find a practitioner experienced in clearing in order to clear the client of outside forces so that you can get accurate answers.

When beginning to work with a client, always set the paradigm so you will know what is "yes" and "no." Generally "yes" is a strong response and "no" is a weak response, but some clients may respond differently. Ask, "Give me a 'yes' and give me a 'no.'" Test twice to make sure you have the right response. If you have been doing muscle testing for many years, you have an indigenous program that sets the basic parameters before you start so you do not have to do any testing. Your basic parameters will followed by the client.

In using Neuro-Kinesiology, you will use both hands. If you ask a question using the arm only, you will be accessing beliefs held in the Conscious Mind, which may not be accurate. Always check to see if the Conscious Mind has a different viewpoint when you begin to do this work so that you can experience the difference. To check Subconscious Mind, put one hand over the solar plexus or third chakra when testing. This will give the Subconscious Mind's viewpoint on the subject. It is always accurate unless you have outside interference. Most forms of Kinesiology suggest that you use light pressure. This may work most of the time but there are occasions when varying pressure must be used due to control by sub-personalities, attached beings or resistance from some program in the mind. Recognizing all the indications that are presented takes practice.

If you begin to test a client whose the arm will not move with any questions, make sure you are not having a muscle battle with a strong person. Explain, "This is not a contest to see if you can stop me from pushing your arm down."

It may take some practice to find just the right amount of resistance to get the three minds to work with the muscles and give accurate readings. If the arm will not go down under normal pressure, you have outside influence. The attached astral beings must be cleared before continuing or they will continue to disrupt accuracy. You may also notice that, at times, the arm will hold, then break and go down. This indicates that the answer would be positive if the person was clear of intervening influences. Finding the controller may take some work, but it must be found or the answers will not be accurate. Sometimes a sub-personality is the cause but, most of the time, it is a hidden attached being. (My book *2011: The New Millennium Begins* gives the process and methods to clear outside attached forces, astral and alien entities.)

When you are asking questions of the Subconscious Mind, accuracy could be compromised by information suppressed in the time-lines, back-up files, denial or denial-of-denial files. The time-line files are written in the year when a traumatic or negative experience happened, and the mind does not want to deal with it. The mind drops it into denial so you do not have to deal with it again. If a lesson has been brought up to deal with and you refuse to acknowledge the lesson, it will be put in denial-of-denial, locked up and will not come up again. It may also have been linked to an autopilot file. If a controller sub-personality was using the program at the time, when it was suppressed on the denial file, the autopilot was also suppressed with it. These must be removed or they will control a person's life.

When all these tests are made, you can be reasonably sure that you can directly contact Higher Self and the Subconscious Mind. If you want to go on-line with the Akashic Internet, then simply connect the phone lines by asking your Higher Self and the Highest Source of your being to connect you. You then can ask questions that are not body-based.

If you choose to use a pendulum, you may run into interference from astral entities, or from entities within yourself or the client. (They can control pendulums without you even knowing it.) It will appear that the answers are correct, but other forces are actually in control. We have experienced this many times over the past 20 years. Because they are heavier, brass pendulums seem to be influenced less. (There are many excellent books in print on pendulums and dowsing. We recommend David Allen Schultz's *Improve Your Life Through Dowsing*, which is available through Personal Transformation Press.)

As with Kinesiology, we must first establish a protocol as to how the pendulum is going swing. Ask your mind to give you the directions for yes and no. Remember the pendulum is just an extension of your mind, and you are projecting the answer out to the pendulum instead of getting it clairvoyantly or through your intuition. Ask it to indicate a no and a yes. The swing will be your guide. Most people will get different to-and-fro and back-and-forth swings or circles. Practice to see what your "yes" and "no" action will be. As you work with the pendulum, you will find there are more answers in addition to yes and no, such as doubtful, not known, etc.

Neuro-Kinesiology uses the same principle. You are getting the information from the client through a muscle reaction instead of using your own intuition. Quite often when working with a client, you will get more accurate answers with muscle testing because you will not be filtering it through your mind that could color the answers if you have strong beliefs, interpretations or feelings about the subject in question.

When we have cleared all outside forces, we must next set up a reasonable understanding with Middle Self that it is not the Source or the phone operator for the Presence of God. Many sub-personalities would like to be in that position, and may well try to convince you of that. In that case, you will be channeling your Middle Self. This will happen when you do not clear it. When you get Middle Self to understand that you sold your power out to it when you were a child due to the need for survival, it will begin to work with you. If it does *not* want to let go of control, you may need to talk with it to bring it around. It might be that it really likes the fact that it can control your life and it feels threatened because it has to give up control. Control sub-personalities may interpret letting go as giving up their power. You may have able to assure Middle Self that it is not losing anything but gaining a new ally because you are reclaiming your personal power. It may glory in the fact that it can manipulate you. If that happens, then all sub-personalities must be deleted from the file before you can claim control. This takes training and experience, so you will have practice this process.

Unfortunately, eliminating sub-personalities does not mean that they are gone forever, because your Conscious Mind can recreate a new set whenever you do not take responsibility to follow through with the decisions you have decided to take action on. Your mind does not like unfinished answers, sentences, actions or commitments you have made. Do not say you are going to do something unless you intend to follow through. If you do not follow through, your mind will assume you did not want to move forward on the decision you made. If you do not take action, your mind has to close that program, so it creates closure by creating a sub-personality and a program about not wanting to take action on that subject. If it happens often enough, then avoider, confuser, procrastinator, disorientor and disorganizer sub-personalities get installed along with a "not wanting to take responsibility" sub-personality. The list can go on and on if you get into indecision and back away from acting on a choice you have made. Any time you make a commitment and do not follow through, a program is created that is interpreted as "I am not willing to take control of my life." If this happens for a number of years, your Instinctual Self will interpret this as if you want to die.

Your mind cannot leave any loose ends unattended; every thought, statement or action you take must have closure; if you start a sentence, Conscious Mind will complete it for you. So every thought and action you create has to be completed or your mind will finish it and file it. It is a very good housekeeper, but it may not complete the task as you would have done.

A program creates a sub-personality and will drive it to get the desired result. If self-rejection is carried to the final stage, it will create a life-threatening illness. There may be disease-specific sub-personalities that were created with the disease, dysfunctional program or belief. A disease, illness or dysfunction cannot exist in the body without a program to drive it. There must be some activating force to break down the immune system or cause stress on the adrenals or the endocrine system. Any form of negative thought or action will start an immediate breakdown in the immune system and the endocrine system. Receptor sites on the leukocytes are notified by the neuro-peptides in microseconds, which begins a physical deterioration of the immune and endocrine systems, which in turn causes the beginning of illness and disease as the immune system function is compromised and fewer T-cells and leukocytes are produced.

When releasing programs, make sure that you check for the sub-personalities that could be enabling them. Each time you clear a time line or operating file, it may activate another series that has been set up to be restored from a back-up file or a denial file.

When clearing karmic files, you must check for gate-keepers, guards and saboteurs that can be connected with the files. They will try to block release of the files. They can be cleared in the same way as attached astral beings.

If a person degenerates or sets up "I want to die" programs, control of the mind/body shifts to the Instinctual Mind. When this happens, programs can be set up in this mind. If there is a conflict in the mind about "I'm afraid to die" and "I want to die," it will set up sub-personalities in the Survival Self, which is part of the Middle Self. This conflict is the main cause of Alzheimer's disease. The two programs cause an Alzheimer's file to be created. This must be cleared before the person begins the backward slide or it will be difficult to stop.

When clearing, you must clear all denial and denial-of-denial programs and sub-personalities. You can bring them up by asking with Kinesiology, "Is this program a belief?" and, "Is this program a reality?" If both are positive, ask Holographic Mind to go through all the veils, shields and illusions in the back-up files, time-line files, the denial and denial-of-denial files, bringing all the hidden files up to the surface to reveal the truth. If the answers continue to come up positive, you have a program that is locked into the physical body. It the "reality" answer comes up weak, then you have a denial. Check for denials and clear them from all files. In cases where the client has been in traumatic situations, time-lines may be in denial files, also. They can also be in autopilot and in denial or denial-of-denial files.

We must also check for reactivator, recreator and regenerator viruses that will create the same program, again and again. These will be attached to individual programs so you must check each program for this each time you clear the program and sub-personality.

We have recently found another program that can recreate sub-personalities and programs. Similar to a computer virus, this program only functions when activated by a word, an activity, a feeling or an emotion. It will activate a program that will run its course and then close down. If you do not catch it during its operational cycle, it disappears. The results or effects of its activity will remain, but we cannot find out how this situation was created until we ask the proper questions to reveal it. We also found another virus that acts the same as a regenerator, which we term an "activator" virus. It can create or activate an existing program that may be dormant.

Each time you clear the sub-personalities will reveal how clients are doing in taking responsibility for their life. Each time they get into a situation where they do not handle it properly and make it a win-win situation, then Middle Self and Conscious Mind will install controller and many other sub-personalities that apply to the situation where the client lost control or did not take total responsibility.

Our mind will reveal our progress in handling our life path by the number of sub-personalities and programs that reoccur over time. Once we clear all the sub-personalities, some will be recreated depending our ability to handle the situations that come up in our life. When we are able to handle all situations without losing our center, needing to be right, being in power and control, giving our power away, and not following through with all our intentions and commitments, then our mind will not install sub-personalities. Anger or resentment will open emotional doors, allowing programs and sub-personalities to be installed. The ideal is to get to a point where no sub-personalities are reinstalled. When this occurs, you will have 100 percent control over your life.

Each time we conduct a session, the controller sub-personalities must be checked. If they keep reoccurring, then we must find out why clients are not taking full responsibility for their life. You may find that they just do not want to take control or discipline themselves. Very few people are actually in control of their life. Many *claim* to be, based on all the seminars, workshops, and therapies they have taken but, in most cases, little has changed.

Taking responsibility is a key issue in everyone's life. Although we had some answers in the past, we could not actually describe how one actually takes responsibility. Now we can, having found all the programs, beliefs and sub-personalities that block a person's ability. (One of the major blocks is plain laziness.) Once we have cleared all the blocks, it is then a matter of the client's *desire*, which is controlled by his or her Conscious Mind. With clients who do not want to apply themselves and step in and become self-actualized, there is nothing we can do as practitioners to change that situation.

We do not judge where clients are on their individual path. Their body/mind reveals that to us. N/CR cannot force them to take control over their life.

Steps Practitioners Must Take Before Beginning Sessions

One of the major mistakes practitioners make is to step into the therapy process without clearing themselves. Practitioners who want to sell you supplements, herbs or drugs, or want prove their point that you need what they are demonstrating to you can do this easily because all people have an authority figure program that gives their power away to people who know more than they do about a subject. We will accept their opinion, which they can prove to us with muscle testing. (There is an affirmation to clear the authority program later in this chapter.)

The tester must be clear of Middle Self control and the need to be right. There are many sub-personalities that will control your ability to use any form of a divination process. The main ones are the Controller, Authority and Manipulator. They always

want to be right. An authority figure can manipulate the test results by the mere fact that the client will give personal power
away to the tester. (This is very common in the medical field.)

If testers are not clear, they will get a desired result to sell the
client their process, a product or to validate themselves. Testers
driven by a sub-personality will not get accurate results. They
must release the controlling sub-personality and reclaim their
personal power. Outside forces can also impose controls on the
effectiveness of testers. They must be clear of attached beings
before beginning sessions or the beings attached to the practitioner will jump over to the client.

In doing this clearing process, testers may run into control or
interference by attached beings. If this happens, you must clear
the entities before going further. You can also have interference if
clients will not identify with the name they are using, and you
should test for name recognition. If the arm goes weak on using a
particular name, test to see which name is causing the difficulty.
Quite often, women will have a negative response to a married
name if they are divorced or separated from their husband. Sometimes, clients can have a negative reaction to the family name if
they had a traumatic childhood. Choose a name that tests positive before testing and test again.

If after considerable testing for name recognition, the tester
is unable to test with muscle testing because the arm will not
move, there is either a power struggle with Middle Self's sub-
personalities or an outside force. It could be that the client does
not know how much resistance to put up during Kinesiology or a
control sub-personality is trying to control. Occasionally we find
that Instinctual Mind is controlling. Quite often we find a possessive being has stepped in, taken over and is controlling the muscle
test. If this is the case, test for entity attachment and clear cords
and entities.

We have an indigenous program that gives away our personal
power to authority figures. It was an acceptable program during
childhood so we would obey our parents, but it has no value as an
adult. This must be cleared, too (see Steps in Sessions below).

Steps that must be followed prior to testing

1. *Ground yourself* and *balance polarity*: This needs to be done only once a day and may be done upon awakening in the morning. This can be done with the wrist-holding process as it provides all the that is needed (see Steps in Sessions). *Do not put shields, robes of color or energy around yourself to protect yourself.* If you do, you will reflect back all the energy and anything you have removed from the person, stopping the effect of healing.

2. *Clear yourself of any attached beings* before beginning a session or you will drop them on a client. Conversely, if you are not protected, clients will drop them on you. One of the major problems we have is passing out in a session caused by entities that will use the client's mental power to knock you out.

3. *Set your paradigm:* Mentally ask the client to give you a "yes" and a "no." Most people will respond with a "no" as weak or down. "Yes" will be strong, or up. Using the fingers (client tries to keep thumb and middle finger together), closed fingers is usually "yes" and weak or open is "no." With the finger method, you can test yourself. The tester can set the paradigm in any manner desired; we prefer "yes" as the arm tests strong, and "no" as the arm cannot resist pressure and becomes weak.

   Have the client hold the arm up and test to make sure it holds up against resistance. Ask the client to say first and last name while you are holding pressure on it, and have him/her continue saying the name until the arm gets weak and goes down. This tests for control by a control/authority sub-personality. Testers can use this test on either clients or themselves.

The most important person to test is the practitioner who is doing the testing. Many times, the tester has received inaccurate answers from me when muscle testing me and wondered why. It is because I know what I am doing and can control the answers but, if the client's sub-personalities are in control, you will not be able to test very effectively. You may want to wait a few minutes and retest to see if Middle Self was playing games. If it is, the arm will resist again. Retest again until the arm becomes weak. The arm may not go down at all. If this happens, then the person cannot function as a tester and get valid results due to control. You must be in a clear space to do effective muscle testing.

One the most troubling issues we find concerns clients who attend the workshops and then begin practicing on others without first working on their own issues. We cannot avoid our own issues, yet we have found that 50 percent of the attendees will not get into recovery. Therapists must be working on their own issues regularly with another therapist, as practitioners must be in recovery working with their own issues all the time. N/CR brings them up and they will interfere with the process when working with a client. If you do not want to work with your own issues, you will slide the client out of the tight space you put yourself in when they come up. You may even pass out during the session if you do not want to face the issue. This can happen to both the client and the practitioner. Sometimes it can happen simultaneously.

Steps in a Session

The following tests must be done in order:
Step 1. Check for Polarity Reversal
Using NK, check polarity. If the arm goes down, polarity is reversed. If the arm is very strong, check for attached beings. If this test yields "yes," then you need to clear entities before going any further. Show the person how to put the wrists together and hold the arms. If it is reversed, a "no" will record as a "yes" and conversely. Restoring polarity can be done using an ancient Chinese balancing method:

Hold your wrists together, with your fingers pointing toward your elbows one on top and one under (which wrist is on top makes no difference). The wrist bracelets at the base of the palms must be touching flat together, so push the offset steps at the base of each palm together. Then hold your hands with your fingers grasping your forearm, pointing toward your elbows just above the wrists and hold for two to ten minutes. For best results, hold for five to ten minutes a day. You will feel your wrist begin to pulse or become warm. Hold until the pulsing stops.

This practice will balance all your electromagnetic fields, your quadrant energies and the electrical flow in the meridians. It will also balance all your chakras and ground you at the same time. Remember that this will not work if the circulation meridian is not connected. The circulation meridian stops at the end of your third or middle finger. When you connect the meridians by holding them together at the wrist, you complete the circuit so that it creates a circular flow of energy around the body. This must be done each day. It will take two weeks to lock it in. It should be continued at least four times a week.

Everyone should do this exercise before getting out of bed in the morning. It takes about five to ten minutes, and balances all the electromagnetic fields, the meridians, quadrant energies and electrical transmission throughout the body.

Sometimes when we get a reading showing a blowout on one side of the body, we have a polarity reversal caused by a birth trauma or a switch of plans before birth where the soul changes the path and chooses different parents than were originally scheduled. They take over a body that would have been stillborn because the original soul had changed its plans and vacated the body before birth. This can be corrected by using an affirmation asking Holographic Mind to erase and delete the file and install a new file to change the polarity balance.

Step 2. Check to see if the client is in body

Using NK, check to see if the client is in the body. (A strong response indicates yes; weak says no.) To pull the client back in, use the following affirmation, asking the client to repeat after you:

"This is _____ (month, day and year). I am _____ (first and last name), I am in my conscious rational decision-making mind."

This will always pull someone solidly back in. You may have to use this during the session, too. Remind the client to use this affirmation every day while doing the balancing exercise in the morning.

If not successful, use the following procedure:

If you get a mushy response after the affirmation, check to see if the client wants to be in the session. There could be fear of having to deal with issues, which will cause the client to block or "gray out." Check for Instinctual Mind control and release that before going any further. You may have to use the affirmation to get the client back into body again. Always finish by stating the name and "I am in my conscious, rational, decision-making mind."

Nowadays, many people are graying out or browning out but don't know it until they are reminded of how it feels. They can function but only at a survival level, so they need to recognize when they are walking out and use the above affirmation (it may be needed 10 or 20 times a day). During a session, if the mind does not want to deal with an issue, it will black clients out. They may appear as if they are going to sleep, but they are actually passing out due to mind control. You will have to bring them back in to the body. Wake them up and ask Holographic Mind to bring them back into the body. This may need to be done numerous times.

Step 3. Opening all files so they can be accessed

We now use an affirmation to open up all the files so we can access them. Quite often we have found that the time-line files are inaccessible and will not be revealed to us unless we open them before we begin reprogramming.

Use the following affirmation to open the files:

"I am asking you, Holographic Mind, to open all files so we can access them now. I am asking you to open Conscious Mind's operating files, Middle Self's files, operating files, Subconscious Mind's operating files, back-up files, and the time-line, denial

and denial-of-denial files. Bring them up to the surface so we can access them now. I thank you for your help."

This opens all files so we do not have to continually check back to see if we are getting all the information from all files.

Step 4. Check for attached beings

I tried to avoid any mention of attached beings for five years after my first experience in 1986, but it kept hitting us in the face. We decided, in 1991, that we had to accept that most people had various forms or beings attached to them. Many people want to believe that they do not exist. At first, even the mention of them scared people. Some people feel that if they do not acknowledge them, they will not bother them. We have found that this is simply not true. We find people describing entities as spooks, boogies, or spirit beings, etc. It makes no difference what you call them. The farther along you are on your spiritual journey, the more you will be waving a red flag because the dark forces are attracted to people who are doing well in their life and try to do anything they can to block that success. Our process is very simple. You do not have to say anything to remove them. You may have to pull cords out before you can continue as they can lock themselves in with cords and implants. Your fingers have etheric extensions up to eighteen inches beyond the end of your physical fingers. Allow your etheric fingers to grab the cord or implant and pull it out.

Study the clearing chapter carefully as there are many forms of entities. The ones we seem to be dealing with most are the rebel Andromedans, which are aliens who have taken over the forth-dimensional dark forces. There are occasional inter-dimensional beings. We must acknowledge that they exist and that there is no way to avoid them. We have no choice and must clear them.

Using muscle testing, ask: "Are there any entities or attached beings, past, present or future, from this or other dimensions or timeframes, in this body, under any assumed names, false identities, masquerades or names that do not identify them, such as ego, High Self or sub-personality?" This will force them to acknowledge their presence.

We discovered the way to clear attached inter-dimensional beings in 1991 during a Level Two workshop. With the client on the table face-up, clap very loudly and quickly over the body, going from head to the feet. After five or six hard loud claps, hit the bottom of the feet (shoes must be off). Move your hands up the client's body to the head, making sure you maintain contact with the body. Some female clients may feel uncomfortable with this process, but we have found if you break contact during the upsweep, the entity will jump back under your hands.

Finally, check with NK to make sure the entities are gone.

The Planetary Commission and Archangel Ariel are assigned the task of "cosmic cops" to assist all spirit beings to the Spiritual Plane. Call on them before you do any release process. If you have problems, call on the White Brotherhood and the Brotherhood of the Light. Ask the White Brotherhood and Ariel's angels to take the entity to the Spiritual Plane, located in the fifth dimension.

This process should not take more than two to five minutes if you do not run into some nasty entities. Don't get caught up finding who they are or carrying on a conversation with them. They have no right to attach to a person's body.

Step 5. Check for AKA cords and implants

AKA cords attach in the third chakra (solar plexus region), the base of the spine, brain stem and sixth chakra (third eye). These are the common locations; they can be at other locations. These generally must be cleared before you can continue with the session as they skew the answers. The cords can have attached beings connected to them and many times the cords or implants will disguise the beings, which must be cleared before you can clear the attached beings.

People in your life who want to control you or leach off your energy can attach cords to you in some of the same areas. At the height of alien activity, we also found many forms of implants, but this has dropped dramatically recently.

Pull the cords with your "etheric fingers." Visualize your fingers with extensions up to eighteen inches beyond the ends of your physical fingers. Allow your etheric fingers to grab the cord or implant and pull it out. (See the implant removal procedure in the clearing section.)

Step 6. Check for Instinctual Mind programs

This is one the most critical dysfunctional programs we are finding now. In the past, I assumed that only people who had serious or life-threatening illnesses had the Instinctual Mind activated. We are finding them on three out five people. In the past we did not check for instinctual files in the average person. You would not suspect them to have them activated. In the fall of 2000, Instinctual Mind files began to show up in everyone as the stress level in society builds up and the pressure shifts as time speeds up as we approach the critical mass shift.

I had just begun checking for Instinctual Mind control and "I want to die" programs, and started to find that they can be activated in anybody. I worked with people who had traumatic experiences in childhood and have had this problem most of their lives although we could not understand the cause. When we cleared the "I want to die" programs, uninstalled the Instinctual Mind, and erased the operating system, it cleared up. If the client feels futility, frustrated, indecision, or loss of direction, the Instinctual Mind program will automatically be installed. Most of the time, *I want to die* and *fear of dying* programs will get installed also. If both of them are installed, you should check for *Alzheimer's* programs as they may be installed, too.

Another aspect we have discovered is that if the Instinctual Mind is able to take over 70 percent control of the mind, it will begin to block out many of the files, such as the love program, file manager, program manager, and sometimes foul up digestive programs, so food will be improperly digested. It will also activate many disorientation and confusion sub-personalities. If it gets 100 percent control, it blanks *all* files. The more control you give it, the more it takes over. If you do not know that it is activated, it will eventually destroy you and you will die or go into regression with Alzheimer's disease.

To clear this program using NK:

i)   Ask: "Are there any instinctual mind files active? How many *I want to die* programs are active? How many *fear of dying* programs are active? Are there any *Alzheimer's* programs active?"

ii) Ask: "Where are these active files? Are they in the: a) Conscious Mind? b) Inner Conscious Mind? c) Middle Self? d) Inner Middle Self? e) Subconscious Mind? f) Backup? g) Denial? h) Denial-of-denial? i) Time-line?"

iii) This affirmation must be for both the *fear of dying* and the *I want to die* programs. To release them, use this affirmation:

"I am asking you, Holographic Mind, to access all files, remove the Instinctual Mind program from Conscious Mind's operating files, Middle Self, Subconscious Mind's files, back-up and time-line files, denial and denial-of-denial files and uninstall the operating system and the operating instructions and put them in the history section. Lock them up so they will not be able to recreate again. Delete, erase and destroy all the programs, patterns and records and the operating instructions and systems. Put them in the archives and lock them up in the recycle bin so they will never affect me again."

"Remove _____ (exact number) 'I want to die' programs and/or fear of dying programs; put them in the archives. Delete, erase and destroy all their operating instructions, operating systems and operating programs, patterns and records. Lock them up in the recycle bin so they will never affect me again. I thank you for your help."

Alzheimer's release affirmation:

"I am asking you, Holographic Mind, to access all files and remove _____ (exact number) Alzheimer's programs and put them in the archives. Delete, erase and destroy all operating instructions, operating systems, programs, patterns and records that

operate the Alzheimer's programs and lock them up in the re-cycle bin."

(Instinctual mind cannot be destroyed as it is an indigenous program.)

From my research, this set of programs is the major cause of Alzheimer's. It really is not a disease, but a shutting down of the mind and a reversal of the growth process. A person is going into retrograde and devolving, going back to birth. You can follow it very well if you watch the person's behavior. As they decline, they will finally go to a point where their organs will not operate and they cannot breath, which is the point of birth and they go bank into the womb. Since there is no support from the mother, their body dies.

Step 7. Make peace with Middle Self and program manager. Make friends with the Ego and File Manager. Reclaim personal power.

Before you can change any programs, you must make peace with Middle Self and take your power back from it. We have to make friends with Ego and forgive ourselves for beating it up. Ask the Middle Self and file manager if they will work with you. Very seldom will we get a "yes" to the question unless the client has done extensive work and has been successful in reprogramming the mind.

Few methods and processes available will be successful in actually reprogramming the mind since they do not first get support from both Middle Self and Ego. Middle Self is the program manager and must work with you to coordinate program installation. In most cases, it was handling writing the programs and installing them. We must take that responsibility back and reclaim our personal power. (This is the primary concept in my books).

Ego is the file manager that files programs in your Subconscious Mind. If it is not working for you, it will not file any programs or affirmations in the Subconscious Mind. The programs must pass through Middle Self's censor program and, if it chooses not to let the file through, affirmations will not work in most cases. If Middle Self is left to run on its own, file manager (Ego) will only install files that Middle Self approves. Middle Self will not give up control since it has been appointed as your protector unless you rewrite its operating system. Ego will not allow programs or files to be installed if it feels that you are attacking it. It is your memory retrieval system so it has to be functioning properly.

Since both program manager and file manager are operating systems, their operating protocol can be rewritten and reinstalled with the proper operating programs. The following affirmations will rewrite the operating systems and the protocol that Middle Self and Ego operate under. They will then cooperate with you and file any program you want them to.

Before beginning any reprogramming, we must use these affirmations:

"I recognize now that I have to make peace with my Middle Self. I know that you are the program manager and you did the best you could with the program you had available at the time. It is my responsibility to reclaim my personal power, and I accept that now. I want you to know, Middle Self, that I am taking my power back now. I am not taking your power. I am only taking back the power that is rightly mine. I have no intention of damaging or destroying you because you are an important part of my team and I need your help. I know I must take my power back and take responsibility for my life now. I let you do that for me in the past. I know that I must be the computer operator and the programmer, and I accept that now. It is my responsibility to install all the program files now. I thank you for your help".

"I want to you to know, Ego, that I have to make friends with you now. I know as the file manager, you did the best you could with the programs you had available to you at the time. Due to false information and a misconception, I felt you were the villain and the enemy. I realize this is a false and erroneous misinterpretation. I know now that you are the file manager, the secretary and the librarian for my Subconscious Mind computers. I recognize my mistake now. I am giving myself 100 percent full permis-

sion to forgive myself for any harm and trauma that I may have inflicted on you in the past. I need your help since you are an important part of my team. I am loving you and forgiving you since I know you did the best you could with the programs you had available. I am loving and forgiving myself. I am installing these operating systems in the file now. I thank your for your help. I am loving and forgiving myself and I am doing that now."

Few practitioners understand or know that these files exist. They wonder why their process does not hold very well. So often, I find people will cling onto the Ego as the controller of their lives even after I prove to them who is doing the controlling. Blaming Ego is so ingrained into our minds that we do not want to let go of the old definition. These two files must be reprogrammed and reinstalled or very little will work over the long haul. Even though this is true for most people, I have worked with clients who were so intent with changing their life that they reprogrammed themselves. The power of the mind is awesome when we get in contact with our own power to work with it.

Step 8. Remove authority figure program

This program gives your power away to authority figures, and is one of the most disconcerting. It was installed as an indigenous program in our mind at birth so we would give allegiance to our parents and follow their guidance as a child. As an adult, it has zero value as it causes us to give our power away to anybody who claims to know more about a subject than we do, be it the plumber, garage mechanic, doctor or lawyer. If a doctor gives us a diagnosis of an illness, even if we do not have it, we will accept the diagnosis and manifest the symptom. We can even pick up something from what we read, hear or see if we give our power away to the authority behind the statement. These all end up as beliefs and will control our life. Quite often, programs that begin to operate from these files can annoy us but we do not know how to change them.

To remove the program, use the following affirmation:

"I am asking you, Holographic Mind, to remove the author-ity figure program. I realize it had value when I was a child so that I would follow my parents' guidance. As an adult, it has zero value as it causes me to give my power away to any person who I recognize as an authority figure. Take this program out of the files and uninstall the operating system. Delete erase and de-stroy all the operating instructions, programs, patterns and records and put them in the archives, locking them up so they will never affect me again. Put them in the recycle bin permanently. Thank you for your help. I am loving and accepting myself now."

Step 9. Check on receiving love

Three out five people are rejected before they are born. Can clients receive love and love themselves? I find very few people are able to love themselves. When looking for these programs, check to see if the mother wanted children in general and if she wanted that particular child. Since I have been checking for the love program over the last 20 years, the statistics have changed. I was not going into the files very deeply at first, so my feedback was that two in five were rejected before they were born. Now it has gone up to nine out of ten. In my work, I can go for months at a time before I find someone who actually loves him or herself. This is independent of age, but I find it children under ten years old are more prone to inability to love themselves.

Check first by using normal Kinesiology using only the arm. Ask the client, "Are you loving yourself and are you receiving love from others?" If the arm goes down, they have no love file, and the mind does not know what love is at all. Sometimes a client may check strong on loving self when it is an illusion be-cause they have been working on themselves for years. They have convinced themselves that they love themselves to the point they will test strong for loving themselves.

If you suspect that this is not true, ask Holographic Mind if this is a belief or a reality. You must have all files open to do so. Check denial files, which may reveal that the first test may be inaccurate.

Remember that this program will not lock the love affirmation into the file unless you release the actual rejection programs that are located in acupuncture points on the body on the left side near the top of the shoulder blade. There are many rejection, "I am not all right," "I do not fit in," "Nobody wants me," "I am not accepted," "Nobody loves me" programs located in the same area if the person was rejected before birth or as a young child.

Use the following affirmation to reinstall the love program:

"I recognize now that love is my responsibility and I accept that now. I know now that I am entitled to unconditional love and I accept that now. I know that love is kindness and caring, acceptance without judgment and control, acceptance without manipulation and authority. I accept that now. I am removing all overshadows that block me off from God and I am doing that now. I know that I can reestablish the presence of God in my life now. I am doing that now. I am removing all inner shadows that block me off from my Higher Self. I am doing that now. I know now that I am entitled to live in peace, happiness, harmony and joy and I accept that now. I am loving myself and forgiving myself and I am doing that now.

This affirmation will rewrite the program every time. The question is, will it continue? If you do not forgive your parents and remove the program from the body files that are located in the area around the shoulder blade on the left side, the love program will be erased and go back to its rejection program again. Just saying the affirmation will not reprogram the file. After you have rewritten the love program, then you can ask why it was lost. We were born with the program intact, but the way we interpret how we were treated after we were born dictates what happens to the program.

Ask the client, "Did your mother want children? Did she want you as a child?"

If yes, continue. If no, then ask, "Did she reject you before birth?"

If yes, then ask, "Did she accept you after birth?"

If yes, continue. If no, then ask, "Did she think about or take any action about abortion?"

If yes, then ask, "Did she ever accept you?"

If no, then ask, "Did your father accept you? Were you the right gender for your parents?"

If you come up with "no" to the last two questions, you have major work to do with the client's forgiveness of the parents. This must be done or the client will never get out of the victim consciousness programs. Some people can pull through without help but only a few. People treat you based on what you project about how you feel about yourself. You will keep drawing people into your life to work these love programs out until you forgive your parents.

Step 10. Release, delete and erase sub-personalities

If time is limited, it is very important to clear the four controller sub-personalities. If you have time, clear all the autopilot and the validation sub-personalities. When you clear them all and you are testing the client in the next session, the number of sub-personalities that have gotten back in will indicate how much responsibility the client is taking to handle and control in his or her life.

Go through the list of autopilot and validation sub-personalities and list the number of each type on the checklist (photocopy the page so you can use each time you do clearing). Check for all virus activators with each file. These will recreate the program or sub-personality after it has been removed (unless they are removed and deleted along with the operating file.) Use the first affirmation to remove all of the sub-personalities. The control sub-personalities must be released before you can work effectively, so first remove them as a group because they will try to interfere if not removed. Then go to the second group. They do not have to be released in the first session. When finished, go to the second affirmation to complete the process.

Sub-personalities

You can delete the programs they have created to support themselves but not the sub-personalities because they are indigenous to the mind, in that they cannot be removed. Quite often people want to blame Inner Child for their problems and separate it from themselves, which is not possible. When someone says, "My Inner Child was hurt," they are trying to avoid responsibility. Inner Child can only record a feeling and/or interpret it, as the Inner Child is part of the mind and is who you are. It may have had to take over working through autopilot, but it has no control over your life when you take responsibility for your behavior. It can only operate through programs that it creates through program manager (Middle Self). When you take your power back and reclaim control of our life, Inner Child grows up and drops out.

In May of 2001, we discovered that Instinctual Self was activating Instinctual Mind by feelings of frustration, indecision, futility and lack of direction. Usually the "I refuse to take responsibility" sub-personality was installed, too. They create *I want to die* programs and *fear of dying* programs.

In the past, we found the Instinctual Mind activated only in people with major traumatic experiences and life-threatening illnesses. But as of the fall of 2000, it seems that they are activated in everyone who feels any of the above feelings or has sub-personalities installed. We are finding Instinctual Mind files activated in three out of five people.

Do not be surprised if you find that some of these sub-personalities number in the hundreds of thousands because they are a build up from birth. In one extreme case, I found over three million external controllers. Very few people have accessed sub-personalities in any form of therapy.

The Five Basic Sub-personalities

These sub-personalities cannot be removed as they are indigenous to your mind and are installed at birth in the Subconscious Mind's files. You can remove the programs and sub-personalities they use to support them, such as addictive, self-pity forms, etc. The five are:

- Survival Self
- Instinctual Self
- Inner Child
- Critical Parent
- Inner Adult.

Autopilot Sub-personalities

These can be installed in all files and all levels of the mind. Write the number next to each one and release as a group. Release these first as a group:

- Power Controller (wants to have power over people, business activities)
- External Controller (wants to control everything around it for security)
- Internal Controller (control over you for security and safety in denial files)
- Internal Controller (in denial-of-denial files)

These must be released, but the time is not as important as the first group.

Justifier	Procrastinator	Feeling of futility
Authority	Confuser	Frustration
Manipulator	Indecision	Saboteur
Resenter	Avoider	Jealous
Self-righteous	Disorientor	Envious
Judger	Disorganizer	Sufferer
Busy-body	Know it all	Won't take responsibility
Struggler	Blamer	I am not all right
Ingratitude	Blocker (causes person to blackout)	

Anger at being rejected and/or abandoned
Anger at not being respected
Anger at not being recognized
Anger at not being accepted

External Validation Sub-personalities:

Empathizer	Savior	Father figure
Protector	Rescuer	Mother figure

Operational Sub-personalities:
Can be located in Middle Self or Conscious or Subconscious Mind:

Nobody Cares For Me		Self-pity
Projector		
Insecurity	Annoyer	Regretful
Nagger	I am unworthy	I am not accepted
I don't fit in	I am not accepted	Feeling sorry for self
Scardy-cat	Liar	Rebel
Lack of trust	Pain addict	Sympathy-puller
God rejects me	Soap opera player	

Wanting other people to make decisions for me
Wanting to be taken care of

Rejection and abandonment sub-personalities can take many forms:
People are rejecting what I say
People are rejecting who I am
Rejection from Mother
Rejection from Father
Rejected by others
People do not trust me
People don't accept me

Anger programs can be supported by many sub-personalities:
These are some of them. You will find more in the clearing process:

Anger at having to reach out   Refusal to step forward
Refusal to reach out   Anger at having to step forward
Anger at moving forward

Fear can take many forms also:

Fear of being rejected   Fear of reaching out
Fear of venturing forward   Fear of vulnerability
Fear of having to take responsibility   Fear being abandoned
Fear of failure   Feeling inadequate

This affirmation is for releasing the following Sub-personalities

1. "As the Christ Master self that I am, I am asking my Holographic Mind and Ego to remove _____ (exact number) subpersonalities and put them in the archives along with all reactivator, recreator, and regenerator viruses. Put them in the archives. Remove, delete, erase and destroy all the operating instructions, operating systems, programs, patterns and records from the operating files. Lock them up in the recycle bin so they will not affect me again."

2. "I am asking you to uninstall autopilot's operating system and put it in the archives. Delete, erase and destroy all the operating instructions, programs, patterns and records and the format that controls and operates auto pilot. Put them in the archives and lock them up in the recycle bin so they will never affect me again."

3. Finish up all sub-personality clearings with (this must be done at the end of each session):

"Empty and clear the recycle bin and make sure all the subpersonalities are removed from all the files in Conscious Mind's operating files, Middle Self's, and Subconscious Mind's operating files, back-up files, time-line files, denial files and denial-of-denial files. Make sure all files are deleted permanently. I thank you for your help."

The following steps are optional and can be done anytime.

Step 12. Check for Vows, Oaths, Allegiances.
Use the following affirmation to release Vows, Oaths, and Allegiances:

"As the Christ Master self that I am, I am now removing revoking, renouncing, rebuking and releasing all vows, oaths and allegiances. (Use the number of and specific vows if necessary.) _____. *I am asking you, Holographic Mind and Ego, to remove all vows, oaths and allegiances, past, present and future, and I am doing that now. Put them in the archives and delete, erase and destroy all operating instructions, operating systems and programs pattern and records. Lock them up in the recycle bin so they will never affect me again. I thank your for your help."*

Step 13. Check for thought-forms (see description sheet)
Use the following affirmation to release Negative Thought Forms:

"As the Christ Master self that I am, I am now releasing all negative thought forms that have been inflicted on me by other people now. I am returning them to the originators for their own deposition with kindness and caring and unconditional love. I am releasing all self-inflicted negative thought forms with unconditional love and kindness and caring and I am doing that now. Delete erase and destroy all the operating programs, patterns and records and put them in the recycle bin so they will never affect me again. I am loving myself and forgiving myself and releasing myself from this bondage now. Thank you for your help."

Step 14. Check for curses, hexes & spells
Use the following affirmation to release Curses, Hexes, and Spells after first checking for the number of each with NK:

"As the Christ Master self that I am, I am asking you, Holographic Mind, to remove _____ *(exact number) curses,* _____

hexes and _____ spells that are affecting me now. We are doing that now. Put them in the archives now. Delete, erase and destroy all the operating instructions operating systems and operating programs, patterns and records. Lock them up in the archives. Remove all reactivator, recreator and Regenerator viruses and programs deleting, erasing and destroying all their operating programs, operating systems and all programs patterns and records. Put them all in the archives and lock them up so they will never affect me again. Thank you for your help."

Step 15. Check financial success, "I am entitled to money and wealth."

"I have accepted that I am not entitled to money, I don't deserve money, I am not able to accept wealth, I can't keep money when I receive it and spiritual people are not entitled to money. These are all false, erroneous beliefs and concepts. I am asking you, Holographic Mind, to remove, delete, erase and destroy these false and erroneous programs, patterns, records, beliefs, concepts, attitudes and interpretations. Put them all in the archives deleting, erasing and destroying all the operating instructions, operating systems, operating programs. Remove delete, erase and destroy all reactivator, recreator and regenerator viruses and programs and put them in the archives. Make sure they are all locked up in the recycle bin so they will not affect me again. Thank you for your help."

Step 16. Correcting the digestive program

People who carry excess weight are not digesting the food that they eat. The digestive system is extracting simple sugars from all the food intake. If people try to lose weight with a protein diet, they will be hungry all the time. When they eat sugar containing food hunger will be reduced. Before any weight reduction is stated this program must be rewritten. If the lack of love program is not corrected, it will be written over and be blocked. If Instinctual Mind is activated, it will block the digestive program. The above programs must be rewritten before the digestive program can be installed.

Ask: "Is your body living on simple sugars?" If yes, then the program must be erased and a new program installed. Use the following affirmation to correct the digestive program:

"I am asking you, Holographic Mind, to remove this defective malfunctioning digestive program that does not allow me to digest protein, carbohydrates, oils, fruits and vegetables. I recognize that I am not assimilating the nutrients from the food I eat. Uninstall this program delete, erase and destroy all the patterns and records, all the operating instructions, operating systems and operating programs. Put them in the archives and lock the up in the recycle bin so they will not function again. I am asking you to install a new digestive program now. I know that I can digest proteins, carbohydrates, oils, vegetable and fruits and assimilate the nutrients for perfect health now. I asking you to install this program in all files now so they will not be tampered with again. Thank you for your help."

Step 17. Sweeping the Back

Begin at the base of the neck where the arms join the body. Sweep your hands, locating aura holes by further testing. Move hands *slowly* down the back, smoothing the aura's magnetic and gravity fields. Do this until the back of the field is smooth. You can test by moving your hand over their field, four to six inches over the back, and feeling where the fields seem to end. They must extend down over the end of the feet. Do the process until this is accomplished.

Step 18. Balance Energy Fields

Have the client sit on edge of table. You sit to their right. Begin with left hand on the back at the base of the spine/first chakra, and the right in front of the body at the same point. Move the left hand up the back, stopping at each chakra, while the energy returns to normal; hold on the occipital points. Bring the right hand up the front, pausing again at each chakra. Hold the forehead and occipital points until you feel they are released.

Step 19. Balance Magnetic and Gravitational Fields

Magnetic and gravitational fields can be lifted or increased by hand movement about the body or head. Fields should be lifted to about six to eight inches over the head. Lift gravitational field in front and back above head. Balance the magnetic field. It should be lifted over the head about eight inches with outside edges over shoulders. Tie off each field by using your hands to lock it in.

Step 20. Pull Up Aura and Wring Out Hands

Sweep up the front and rear of the fields one or more times, wringing out the hands as a final balance and to pull off anything you might have left there. This also breaks your connection to the client.

If we are going to provide effective healing, we cannot protect ourselves with robes or shields of energy or color. These will protect us, but will also reflect all the dysfunctional energy patterns we are trying to release right back to the client. We must be willing to take on any energy, disease, illness or dysfunctional pattern to release it from the client. It is not in our karmic pattern to have that in our body, so it will pass through us and be discharged into the earth. There has to be an end deposit of any energy. If you throw it out into air or discharge it without a known end point, it can stick on someone without their knowledge.

During treatments or your daily routines, *you* may pick up emotional or physical sludge that needs to be released. To do this, sit with your feet on the ground (preferably in water, such as a hot tub). Ground yourself with the roots. Let earth energy run up the roots to the top of your head. Then, allow white light to come down and fill your body the same way, visualizing it flowing into your body down through the crown, all the way to your feet. Bring the "Pacman" out of your head and visualize him cleaning out your body by gobbling up the garbage as he moves through your body. Allow him to move through your body until he has gone through every muscle, cleaning it of all the loose energy or garbage you may have picked up during the day. Right above your base chakra, visualize a canister to deposit the garbage. Blow it down the roots when finished. When completed, run energy again from head down and from ground up to refill, balance and ground again. If you get up quickly after doing this process, especially if you've dumped a lot, you may feel dizzy or pass out. Let yourself balance out before standing up.

Step 21. Empty the recycle bin

At the end of each session, make sure you clear the recycle bin and empty it. Delete all the files that have been put there during the session.

Affirmations Used In sessions

Affirmations, the Software

Affirmations are the backbone of N/CR as they are the software that we use to rewrite the programs. The practitioner cannot rewrite the programs. No matter how hard you try to convince the client's mind to accept the affirmation, it will not always do this. The only person who can do this is the client. Nobody can reprogram you without your permission. You have to accept the programming. If you are not in control of your mind, a therapist can make a diagnosis or tell you have something and your mind will accept the belief if you have an authority figure program by which you give your power away to people in authority.

N/CR is a right-brained, feeling level process. We always ask clients to get into their feeling level and not analyze the process. You may find some clients have resistance to following you in repeating the affirmations. If this happens ask them to help you in forming the affirmation.

Affirmations are the key to effectiveness of N/CR. They are the way we talk to the Middle Self, Ego, Subconscious, Holographic and Intellectual Mind to get them to support releasing negative energy from the body. The purpose of this section is to reveal how effective affirmations are structured and the purpose of each part of the affirmation. As you will find, keeping these general structures in mind will speed your work and give you confidence in your own abilities. N/CR would not work effectively without affirmations. You can hold points for minutes to hours, which will achieve energy releases but no more. You must locate the base cause, core issue and sometimes the catalyst, then release the pattern and programs to release the dysfunctional program. Releases should take about 30 seconds to a few minutes.

Often however, the body you are working on will give you different affirmations than the ones listed here. Sometimes, you will find that you are not even using the standard format. This is perfectly fine because we are really interested in obtaining release of subconscious negative programs and improving the thought processes of the Conscious Mind. Go with whatever works! Do not feel you have to follow the affirmations given in this book. Let your mind form the affirmations that apply. The patterns listed here are an excellent, proven way to start, and you may find that, when you get very comfortable with the process in general, you will decide to stay with this general format. You will find that, after some practice, you are forming your affirmations as you go. There is no need to memorize affirmations. This will take some practice and trust in yourself that you can do it. Once you make a win-win situation for yourself by letting yourself open up to the concept that you can do it, they will begin to flow very easy.

The General Pattern for Affirmations

The general pattern we use is a simple four-step affirmation. If you want to work further with affirmations for any purpose, you will find this format to be an effective one for almost all situations. The four steps are done in order to logically satisfy the intellectual mind and to build a strong case for internal support.

The four steps are as follows ("you" refers to the client):

1. Acknowledge who you are and claim your power
2. Acknowledge your creation of a situation, and release …

3. Release person, situation or anything else involved
4. Release yourself.

Let's look at each step in more detail to see what they are about and why they are included where they are, as opposed to anywhere else in the process, or not included at all.

1. Acknowledge who you are and claim your power
This step is first because you must call upon your inner powers to direct the energy. If you do not first claim your power, you cannot do anything. This is one reason why many affirmations do not work. Energy is not power! Power is the ability to command energy, while energy is what gets the work done. We usually use the phrase, "As the Christ Master self that I am ..." to satisfy this part of the affirmation.

You may need to adjust the phrasing or the name you call the Christ Within in case you are dealing with someone not raised Christian. In this case, use whatever name they supply to you, but it is important that they get in touch with the name of the presence of the deity with which they were raised as that is the name the Middle Self identifies with power.

If you work on an atheist, you can substitute something like, "As the Awakened Consciousness, Powerful Being that I am ..." or something similar. If in doubt, ask clients how they address their most powerful self. After a few sessions, you may find it possible to switch to the current representative of God. Just be absolutely sure that the entity you are calling on to help is a true ascended master, and not some guru or impostor. Watch for the Middle Self addressing itself, too. We have found the process works with people who claim to be atheists also. But, they must have strong convictions of who they are and have some understanding of love as it applies to them.

We have found that since you are working with a computer, saying, "I recognize now", or, "I am calling on my Holographic mind to help me," will be accepted by the mind. So, we do not put a lot of emphasis on the preamble as in the past. We have used the affirmations without any phrase to acknowledge the presence of a Source of God within and it seems to work very well.

2. Acknowledge your creation of the situation, and release ...

When you are talking to the Subconscious Mind and it responds without resistance, we have no problem. We are using the preamble to the affirmation to help clients claim their personal power. In actuality, the mind works like a computer, so we can use very short affirmations. There is no need to get into elaborate strung out affirmations. All your Subconscious Mind wants to know is:

1. Are you willing to accept that you participated in the event?
2. Are you going to release blame and accept that what happened "is what is."
3. Are you going to forgive and love the person and/or the event?
4. Are you willing to accept that you are all right no matter what happened?
5. Are you going to release and forgive and love yourself?

This is all you need do to release any dysfunction from the body. The body/mind will take care of everything else that is required for healing. We do not use flowery, metaphysical-based affirmations, since we are working with an analog computer that is very linear in its concepts.

When we discovered that the mind backs up all programs daily, it opened a new vista in getting to the cause of why some patterns did not release or were recreated and were restored to the file. We recently found that the mind or outside forces can set up activator or recreator viruses that will rewrite the same program that is in a back-up file.

Files may often be covered up so they will not be revealed on the first release. Then they will come up later as the computer will fill the empty file space with a program or a pattern that was below it in the file.

We have found that many times we have had to go through all the files to release a program. Each level of the mind may contain the same file if it was a traumatic experience. Sometimes the file may be buried in denial or denial-of-denial.

Recently, we have discovered another level that we knew existed but never examined it. We are finding many connections to programs in the future time-line file. This file will set up a program to activate on a particular date in the future. If we can access them before they happen, we can avoid considerable problems that may come in the future. Quite often they are connected to existing programs that have been suppressed in denial and/or denial-of-denial files.

3. Release person, situation or anything else involved

The descriptive part is the situation or what happened that caused the breakdown or dysfunction.

4. Release yourself

The closing must include a statement forgiving and loving the person involved in the situation and loving and forgiving yourself.

Individual affirmations may be as long as twenty minutes in length if there is resistance to rewriting by the client's belief structure. Quite often, a sub-personality is holding onto the program. Open doors from past lives may also need to be cleared. The blocks that will stop the reprogramming are denials and denials-of-denials. If they are present, the client may not know that the program or belief exists or may deny that this is their problem. These must be cleared before we can continue.

Sometimes emotions will surface in the form of crying or some other cathartic release. This will not release the program but it does release pent up feelings and energy.

I no use longer hypnosis to access past lives as I feel it is less effective and takes too long. I have also found that I am often unable to get the client to regress to the life we need to experience to release the situation. Instead, I use an affirmation to bring up the file so that we can view it.

If I can get the file directly from the client, I use it, otherwise I go to the Akashic Record and ask for the file. We can't do that in hypnosis if the file is blocked from the client's mind.

Viewing past lives takes clairvoyant ability. I have found that some people will be able to pick up the past life just by saying the affirmation.

Occasionally a client will auto-regress and actually re-experience the lifetime we are examining, in which case, I ask questions to guide them through it.

The affirmation I use is:

"As the Christ Master self that I am, I am releasing myself back to my original incarnation to review all records, patterns and programs in reference to _____ [insert situation]. I am bringing them up to the present time so we can review them now. I am now bringing them up to the present moment to we can release them now. I am doing that now."

Let the file come and view it.

The closing affirmation I use is:

"I recognize now that I can release this _____ [incident]. I am claiming grace now. I am totally committed to releasing this now. I am asking you, Holographic Mind, Ego and Subconscious Mind, to take these patterns, programs and records out of the file. Delete, erase and destroy all of the operating instructions, all of the programs, patterns and records and put them in the archives. Lock them up so they will not be able to activated again. So they will not be accessible by me or anyone else. I have claimed grace now. I thank you for your help. I am loving myself and forgiving myself knowing this is locked up now."

Closing Remarks

The process clears clients so that they do not influence the outcome of muscle testing. If the Middle Self's control sub-personalities have to be right, they will influence the outcome of any process. With a few clients, I have never been able to get them clear because the denial sub-personalities and the auto-pilot had total control. The vast majority of clients, however, can be cleared.

Have clients hold an arm out. Apply constant pressure on it while they repeat their first and last name. Increase the pressure while the clients repeat their name until the arm weakens and you can push it down. Try it a second time. If there is no resistance, then the person is clear. If clients refuse to let you check for clarity or are defensive, know that you will not receive accurate answers from them.

Chapter 16

Afterthoughts and Conclusion

What 20 years ago we described as Structural Integration is now termed "psychoneuroimmunolgy" by the medical establishment, yet I doubt that they really know what they are describing. (Doctors routinely name something and then chase its symptoms until they find out what it really is and how to work with it.)

Over the years, the effectiveness of N/CR has increased steadily thanks to feedback from clients and workshop participants. The process has shifted from a totally body-based focus to a combination of kinesiology and mind-reprogramming with affirmations to release beliefs and denials that are run by sub-personalities.

We continually upgrade the technique to make it more effective, to the point that now, there is no illness, disease or behavioral dysfunction that cannot be treated. If clients will cooperate and commit themselves to healing, we have the tools to create perfect health with unconditional love, peace, happiness, harmony, and joy with financial abundance.

In the beginning, situations would come up that I did not understand; we would release programs and patterns yet the condition would persist or return. What we did not know was that if we didn't clear the beliefs about the situation, then the belief would simply create a new program and maybe a new sub-personality that would in turn create a habit pattern. Further, if clients denied the behavior, they would also create a denial sub-personality. And since the mind is program-driven, all action we take will result in some form of programming to the database.

Psychological training routinely includes Transactional Analysis, which although it identifies many sub-personalities, does not locate all of them. We have identified over 35 sub-personalities, many of them covered up by denials of the dysfunctional behavior they are driving. This major find opened up the final phase in understanding human behavior by confirming that allergy/health dysfunction syndromes have no physiological basis and do not respond to drugs, yet they can be cleared and healed with reprogramming.

Another common problem is that clients will not stick with the process long enough to complete the therapy process. Some fear or other will come up thanks to a denial sub-personality and that ends the process. The clients will not see the fear that is driving them to separate from clearing the programs. While unfortunate, I cannot control clients' behavior, nor would I want to.

Enlightenment and transformation can take many lifetimes if people drag their feet, are fearful of vulnerability, and want to justify and blame. The only road to transfiguration is love, forgiveness and acceptance. That does not mean giving up your personal power or your freedom. It means that you must recognize the lesson in every situation and take the path that leads to further transformation without playing victim or placing blame. We create *all* the lessons and situations in our lives, so all we need do is validate ourselves and recognize that no one hurts us unless we let them do it. *The only person who rejects you is you.*

Many times, when my clients reclaim their personal power, they become arrogant and aggressive. While this is not the proper path, if they are coming out of a lifetime of victim consciousness, the resentment is often still programmed in the files. I have often seen covert control starting to come up in clients who are not willing to take their power back, so they are continuing their victimhood by controlling behavior. Assertiveness does not mean taking advantage of, or walking over someone else. It means being aware of how you present yourself and standing up for yourself.

Meta-communication will always reveal your actual feelings and reactions to any given situation. Body language and non-verbal communication is not limited to visual cues. Being able to read between the lines of the spoken word also reveals how a person feels. The construction of written sentences also reveals their actual feelings.

We can twist anything around to overlay it with the interpretation we want, and if we are in denial and deluding ourselves, we will assume that the recipient of what we say or write shares our intentions and motives. However, if you are aware and observant, you can read between the lines and detect the recipient's real feelings. When you read a book or a letter, you can actually tune into the writer's unwritten thoughts and feelings. I have often experimented by reading a book and then asking others to read a certain page. Frequently, they cannot discern the same information that I had seen on the page in my mind's eye.

We have to be very careful what we say and what we write. Your body is constantly talking. *Are you listening?*

Appendices

Appendix A: N/CR Questions and Answers

Q: What comprises an N/CR Session?

A: We will be working with Neuro/Cellular Reprogramming, Behavioral Kinesiology, and biofeedback, if necessary. We demonstrate methods to understand the dialogue, misperceptions, and interpretations that the Subconscious Mind has stored in its memory. The acupuncture points on the body are switches or gates. Putting pressure on these entry points turns on the mind's "VCR" and opens the dialogue with the Subconscious Mind's files.

We must resolve certain basic issues before we can begin the process:

1. The client must be anchored in the body. Many people are out of their body and are unaware they are not functioning in their body, especially if they are confronting a traumatic issue. However, once they know how it feels, they can recognize when this has happened.

2. Electrical polarity must be correct in order for Kinesiology to work properly. If the polarity is reversed, "yes' will appear as "no" and "no" as "yes." We cannot obtain an accurate answer until polarity is balanced properly.

3. Therapists must allow themselves to be loved and love themselves. Separation from Source will cause a lack of love, along with self-rejection. We must accept our entitlement to love.

4. We must find out if the three lower minds are going to work with us. If not, then we must rewrite and reprogram the tapes. We must get Ego to recognize that we are not going to destroy it, and to convince it to be our friend.

At this point, we are now ready to ask questions with Kinesiology, or go directly into program releases. We can go directly to the root causes and the core issues stored in the Subconscious Mind's files. This will reveal the programs that have become habit patterns that are causing dysfunctional behavior, illness, diseases or pain in any form. We can release and heal any dysfunctional program in a very short time with use of Neuro/Cellular Therapy.

I recommend taping all sessions for the protection of both therapist and client. Also, the session can be reviewed and transcribed. There will be many parts of the session the client will not be able to recall because the mind may block it out. Many people have found that repeating the affirmations will lock in the new programming.

Q. Why is this particular process so effective?
A. Unlike other therapy processes, the client is required to participate in the session. The client is not *worked on*. In most treatments, such as Rolfing, Trager, massage, acupuncture, and other body-related processes, you do not participate. In psychology, you will be asked what your problem is, but few clients know what the base cause is, so how can we work with a belief, concept, or a program when we are not sure of the cause? The body will always reveal the base causes and the core issues if we listen to it.

We have to get Middle Self to cooperate with us, as it is one of the main players in the game. The Middle Self knows exactly what is happening in our life, so we need its support. All levels are brought in to play, physical, emotional, mental, spiritual and etheric, all at the same time. The body being a hologram, we access all levels of the mind and body with Kineseology and with clairvoyance to access the records that we need in releasing the programs. We go one further by accessing the ability of the Higher Self.

Q. What should you expect during a treatment?

A. To understand what a treatment is like, you must first understand what it is not like. No special preparations or clothing are required. You will not experience any deep tissue work that is painful, nor will you be required to accept altered states of consciousness. We do not use hypnosis or guided imagery. You will not expected to dredge up painful, emotional experiences from the past or "lead the discussion" as in analytical psychology. In fact, you do not need to tell us anything. Your body will reveal all we need to know, although we may ask some questions to establish some basic criteria.

Emotions may come up and you may experience flashbacks during the process but they are all momentary and release quickly.

We use affirmations as the means to reprogram and rewrite scripts in the mind. The therapist creates the affirmation, then the client repeats the affirmation. The only person that can reprogram your mind is you; there is no such person as a healer of others. You can only heal yourself. As such, we are only facilitators to direct the process.

Q. What goes on during a treatment?

A. When we locate the cause or core issue with kineseology, we must determine if it is a belief or reality. If it's only a belief, it may be controlled by a sub-personality. In either case, we can release it with an affirmation that will reprogram the software. If it is body-based, then we have to locate the acupuncture point that holds the incident we are releasing; a momentary pain will occur at that point. As we bring up details of the incident and forgive the cause, it will disappear immediately.

We do not experience the mind's action during the process; it instantly communicates to the body through neurosynapses and signals the muscles to let go of the tension. At the same time, it is rewriting the programs in the computer. Through affirmations, we communicate what we want to happen. It is important to understand that you are giving permission and removing the programs yourself. As the therapist leads you through the affirmation, you are healing your own body. The therapist is actually just a facilitator who has agreed to let you release the negative energy through him/her, providing an opportunity to experience love and forgiveness to release the incident.

Q. How long does this take and how much?

A. The number of treatments depends on your willingness to let go. Taking responsibility to see life differently without judgment, justification, rejection or fear/anger helps. A typical average is three to ten sessions. Some clients have had over 100 sessions, while others have cleared most of their issues in four to ten. There have been miracles in one session, but they are rare.

The cost of a session is $75/hour, and typically lasts about 80 minutes. Call (800) 655-3846 for an appointment. If you are interested in spreading the word of this work please call us. We would be happy to work with you.

Q. How can I become a sponsor?

A. We teach the Neuro/Cellular Repatterning process in a five workshop series. If you would like to help us present lectures or introductory workshops, please call the number above. We provide a free session if you set up a lecture for us (a minimum of ten people). If you are interested in setting up appointments for me at a designated location I will provide you with a free session for each day I work at your location. (there is a minimum number of session each day to qualify)

Appendix B: The Body/Mind Harmonizer: A New Concept for the New Millennium

Disclaimer:

The following description is of an experimental device intended for research in electronic medical experiments. We are not medical doctors or psychiatrists and make no medical claims or prescribe or diagnose any ailment, illness or disease. Due to FDA regulations we cannot make any claims as to what these devices will accomplish. Following is a report on the results of our research.

The Harmonizer Concept

The physical body matches itself to the frequencies in its environment, whether stressful or not. The Harmonizer counteracts the stress in its immediate vicinity, allowing the body to come into earth resonance, which is the most effective frequency for the endocrine system to balance and regenerate itself. The coil-antennae produces a scalar wave field pulsing on and off to create the effect. Technology for the Harmonizer was developed in the early 1900s by Nikola Tesla, who did considerable research into electromagnetic fields and their generation by special coils. He discovered the so-called *scalar field*, a longitudinal wave field that functions outside the space/time of our third-dimensional world. Since it operates beyond space/time, it is unencumbered by the limitations of conventional physics, and is the most effective way to protect the body from disruptive stress of disharmonic fields or vibrations.

We have also found that earthbound spirits, alien entities and extraterrestrials cannot handle the frequencies, and cannot attach to a person in the Harmonizer's field. The scalar wave radiation also blocks abduction and protects from psychic attack.

People who have been harassed by earth-bound spirit beings have reported that they have been free of them as long as they keep the unit on them 24 hours a day. This was primarily why we developed this unit. Now we find that it does much more than we expected.

The Harmonizer causes accelerated healing up to ten times the norm, apparently by activating cellular restructuring in the body. Generating a high-frequency bio-electrical field using Tesla technology, the unit reportedly accelerates healing at the cellular level, balances the endocrine system, supports the immune system, rebuilds bone structure, and heals skins cuts and lesions about ten times faster than normal. It also seems to balance the electrical function in the body, which in turn can balance all electrical aspects of the body including blood pressure and neurological function.

The Harmonizer Theory

When it is in perfect health, every living being resonates at its own characteristic frequency. Each component of that being's body also resonates at a particular frequency, and if subject to higher frequencies from its environment, it tried to match those frequencies, which causes stress, and that particular cell, organ or gland is weakened, making it more prone to disease or illness.

A tuning fork in the field of another matched fork that is struck will vibrate at the same frequency. Your body does the same thing. When you are subject to negative vibrations such as stress, fear, or anger in your environment, you begin to identify with this environment and your body begins to resonate with that vibration.

If you go into flight or fight, your adrenals kick in, causing a strain on the immune and endocrine systems. A strong dose of adrenaline helps you handle the perceived danger. Under normal circumstances, when the danger is over, your body should release a shot of nor-adrenaline as an antidote so you can return to normal energy and frequency level of 12 – 18 Hz. But, if you live in perpetual stress, survival fear or confrontational conditions, your body frequency will rise to 250 – 550 Hz, over *thirty* times higher than it should be. As your body frequency rises, you begin to function on adrenaline alone.

Electronic devices that emit strong fields also interact with the physical body's electric and electromagnetic fields. The body/mind will identify with the frequency that has the strongest effect on it. The Harmonizer creates a 15-foot diameter field of energy around the body that blocks out other frequencies that are stressful to the body. It emits a low frequency—the Earth resonance signal—and a high frequency that is the ideal frequency for the body's functioning.

The brain's chemicals, such as interlukens, seratonin, interferon, etc. operate at the Earth resonance 12 – 15 Hertz. The immune system and the endocrine system work more effectively when there is no load on the adrenal glands. Negative sensory input or negative thoughts and emotions cause the neuropeptides to slow down, compromising the immune and endocrine systems.

The body's natural electrical field (chi, ki or prana) must be strong to ward off disease factors, but as its frequency rises, the electrical and auric fields weaken, and offer less protection. The Harmonizer causes the mind to focus its energy and operate at optimum health. However, the device is only an adjunct to such measures as proper nutrition. You cannot abuse or mistreat your body and expect the Harmonizer to overcome this.

The following is a greatly simplified explanation of the theory behind the Harmonizer. The information that regulates the various parts of the body is carried by the body's neurological network system. The brain serves as a "switching center" that directs the electrical impulse information and neuropeptides through the meridian system network to the appropriate parts of the body.

Each cell is a mini "computer" in this network, and receives its orders from the mind through the neurological system, carried by electrolytes and the neuropeptides. When operating properly, the cells maintain a delicate balance of chemicals. When they go out of balance or get run down, the electromagnetic fields break down or blow out. The cell loses its ability to protect itself properly. The brain/mind's ability to communicate with the cellular computers breaks down and the body becomes subject to attack by diseases, illness and outside forces, and ***accelerated aging***— the most damaging effect of increased stress and high frequency.

The results are illness, depression, chronic fatigue, emotional instability and life-threatening disease. Metabolism is affected due to breakdown of the function of the endocrine glands, and the body's absorption of nutrition is impaired.

As the body's internal frequency rises past 50 Hz, the good "happy" brain chemicals shut down and the adrenals kick in larger doses of adrenaline to keep you functioning. The adrenals become overworked, which leads to adrenal insufficiency. When production drops below 30 percent, normal fatigue sets in, similar to low blood sugar tiredness caused by hypoglycemia.

Continued high frequency interference causes breakdown in all systems of the body, resulting in Chronic Fatigue and Epstein-Bar Syndromes, which lead to clinical depression. Many doctor prescribe Prozac, Zolov, Valium or other mind-altering anti-depressants, which can be addictive because they suppress the symptoms and fool the brain into believing that the total body malfunction is a false message.

Low Frequency Operation

The Harmonizer balances electrical, metabolic and electro-magnetic system dysfunction by shutting out the disharmonious stress that causes the body to elevate its frequency. It emits a fifth-dimensional etheric scalar field that strengthens all the systems of the body by bringing down the frequency to the optimum level for perfect health.

To be in balance, most devices, plants and animals have clockwise and counterclockwise positive and negative energies. A few plants such as garlic, onion, and some herbs radiate a double-positive field, hence their antibiotic healing qualities. The Harmonizer also radiates a double-positive field, which explains the response it creates.

For more than 200 years of recorded history, the Earth's resonant frequency or Schumann Resonant Factor was 7.83 Hz but, recently, it has risen to 12 – 14 Hz. Our original Harmonizers were built to emit 7.83 Hz, and later models have kept pace with the Schumann frequency. The current 12.5 Hz field helps the adrenals to heal and resume their normal operating level. At this ideal frequency, all organs and endocrine glands function at their most effective level and your body begins to heal because when the body is in the Harmonizer's 15-foot diameter field for a period of time, it will match the Harmonizer's frequency. This may take up to three days depending on your body, but you will notice your body begin to slow down and relax.

High Frequency Operation

The unit also emits a high frequency of 9.216 MHz. When we began our search for the high frequency that would accomplish our purposes, we checked through hundreds of frequencies. Little did we know that the frequency we finally choose was only 0.02 MHz off the actual frequency of the Ark of the Covenant. Apparently, this is a universal frequency that will activate the body's healing modalities and repel anything or anybody who emits a negative energy.

Initially, we were able to get 9.216 MHz chips because Motorola had over-ordered but we have since found other readily available sources. For the latest model, we redesigned the entire circuitry and coil, and used a slightly larger case to accommodate the rechargeable battery pack. As a result, the unit now has a much lower power requirement and is more effective.

When we discovered that we were getting a scalar wave without the circuitry to produce it, we asked some experts about it. All they could say was, "You're dealing with hyper-dimensional physics and it's over our heads and we can't explain it. This is Tesla and Einstein's realm, and we don't understand what's happening."

We are apparently producing an output that no one understands. Nor has any history of this effect been recorded. Two new research consultants joined our team—a radio frequency engineer and a physicist— and they said, "As far as we can tell, it appears that we're on the threshold of a new discovery in quantum physics. We can't measure the scalar field output because it's outside conventional physics, but the radio frequency seems to be a carrier wave for the scalar field."

Harmonizer History

Our first prototype had a weak field, yet it worked so well that we knew we were on to something so we continued our research. The second generation unit had a 100 millivolt output, and the current production unit puts out 800 millivolts. The first unit of the current (tenth) generation had a metal core coil that was absorbing two thirds of the output, so our engineer suggested using a nonreactive plastic core. When we went to a nylon core, we discovered that power output tripled. The next challenge is to build an even more powerful unit that will not interfere with short wave or TV reception, or we would run into trouble with the FCC.

The device uses a triple-wound bifilar toroidal coil/antenna driven by complex electronics that were not available in Tesla's time. Today's computer chip technology has allowed us to reduce the size of the original prototype by over 90 percent. The first generation prototype had a range 18 inches and a battery life of 80 hours. The second generation had a range of 3 feet and a battery life of 260 hours. Early units used expensive 9-volt batteries, and we switched to AA Nicad rechargeable battery packs that lasted about a year. Today's tenth generation has a range of 15 feet and a nickel hydride battery pack that lasts up to four years.

Warning:
Charge the unit for one hour a month, or four hours if it is fully discharged. This is very important, as we have had people return the unit, complaining that battery would not charge. They had over-charged the battery for many hours.

When you first begin to use the Harmonizer, you may find that it needs to be recharged more often than once a month. If your body energy is low and you have been under considerable stress, this will drain the batteries more quickly as the unit interfaces and responds to your body energy level. We have had reports that people have had to initially charge the battery as often as once a week.

Testimonials

Disclaimer: Due to FDA regulations, we make no claims as to what the Harmonizer can accomplish. However, we can report what users have relayed to us. Many claims have been made by users of the Harmonizer but we can not recommend it for anything as we are not psychiatrists or doctors. We are not allowed by law to diagnose or prescribe.

Here, we relay the experiences of those who have used the Harmonizer. For example, many people have reported that it pulled them out of depression in 5 – 14 days without any drugs, and many have ceased taking prescription antidepressants. Two psychiatrists validated this information from their experience.

In my case, I injured my foot with a chain saw, and the wound was not healing well but, as soon as I began using the new Harmonizer, my foot began to heal at an unprecedented rate. I could actually see it heal from one day to the next. The deep gash closed up and healed over in less than two weeks, and today has left only a faint red mark.

1. "It seems to bring programs to the surface that I had no awareness of. It's the best therapeutic tool I have come in contact with." *B.E., California*
2. "I strapped the Harmonizer over a broken leg on the cast where the break was and the break healed four times faster than normal. The doctor was amazed that we could take the cast off in less than four weeks." *J.S., California*

3. "Chronic Fatigue I'd suffered for years disappeared in less than a week." *J.C., Arizona*

4. "I am feeling general well being and able to handle stress more effectively. I'm not getting angry as quickly as in the past. One day, I left the Harmonizer at home and I noticed my stress level began to rise at work." *C.D., California*

5. "Psychiatrists who have purchased the Harmonizer report that it works with depression very well since it reactivates the brain chemicals and supports the rebuilding of normal production of all the essential brain chemicals, allowing the adrenals to slow down and heal. As a result people seem to pull out of depression." *R.N., Virginia*

6. "I put the Harmonizer on a plant that was dying, and it revived in just one day." *T.K., California*

7. "A burn totally disappeared in three days. This was apparently caused by the activation of the cellular restructuring." *J.T., California*

8. "It apparently has caused my immune system to rebuild because I am recovering from a long term illness. It is feels great to get my stamina back." *W.B., New Mexico*

9. "It activates programs in the mind that have been covered up for years. Apparently denial programs are forced to the surface." *H.M., California*

10. "I am finding I have more energy and I sleep less now that the stress is relieved." *G.B., Colorado*

11. "I have been taking drugs for depression, and low thyroid and adrenal function. I continued to take the drugs until they ran out. I noticed that I was getting the same effect from the Harmonizer so I did not renew my prescriptions. That was three years ago and I have not had any depression since. And the new Harmonizer is even better. Thank you so much." *A.P., California*

12. "I handed the unit to friend of mine and he dropped it immediately, saying he couldn't hold onto it. Once I cleared him of attached entities, he had no problem holding it." *J.O.E., California*

13. "I had been to the doctor for my high blood pressure and he prescribed medication to control my blood pressure because it was 190 over 120. I checked it again a month later and it was

still the same. I bought the Harmonizer and started carrying it with me all the time. Less than a month later, I was down to 120 over 70. The doctor could not understand how my blood pressure would come down to normal. 'That just does not happen to someone your age.' I cannot attribute it to anything other than the Harmonizer." *C.S., Arizona*

14. "It is amazing. I felt burned out and the doctor said my adrenals were very low and wanted me to take drugs to build them back up. I told him I did not take drugs of any kind and would find another way. I started using the Harmonizer, and my adrenals recovered in three days. I do not feel as stressed out anymore. This is truly electronic medicine." *K.S., Oregon*

15. "I have had a umbilical hernia for 25 years, and have consistently refused surgery to repair it, instead doing exercises to strengthen the abdominal muscles so it would repair itself. It had been slowing getting smaller, but very slowly. I had the earlier version of the Harmonizer for four years and while it helped in many ways, it had no effect on the hernia. But with the new high frequency unit, in just three months the hernia has reduced to about one quarter of what it was last year." *A.M., California*

16. "My husband had flu twice this winter and I usually get it from him and end up down for a week. This year, no flu or anything. I can only assume the Harmonizer protected me and kept my immune system up to par so I was not affected." *C.H., California*

17. "For me, the Harmonizer is a miracle because I seem to go out of my body quite often and driving is very dangerous when this happens. I have been solidly in my body since I have been using the Harmonizer." *J.S., California*

18. "I have had serious immune system problems for years. It seems that I catch everything that comes along. The Harmonizer has upgraded my immune system to the point that I am now very seldom sick." *C.K., California*

19. "When I called to find out about the unit, I was willing to try anything as my blood pressure was 210 over 120 and I had lung congestion. My legs hurt so much I could not even walk around the grocery store. In five weeks my blood pressure

dropped to 130 over 90 and still continues to fall. I have no lung congestion and I can drive trucks again. I have gone back to work full-time."

20. "As a healer, I touch many clients in my work and would frequently have entities attaching to me from my clients. Today, I would not be without my 'boogie buster' because it protects me so well." *J.N., California*

21. "I have had low adrenal function almost all my life. Stress really takes me down to the point where I can't function. With the Harmonizer, I have recovered totally. I have not experienced any depression or lack of energy since I began using it." *C.K., Colorado*

22. "Accelerated healing of burns has been amazing. I spilled boiling water on my face when I dropped a teakettle. The burn marks began clearing up in two weeks. In a month, they were almost gone except for redness on the skin. Today, there is no scarring and all the marks are gone." *M.K., Arizona*

23. "One of the most amazing results I have found from using the Harmonizer is that old burn scars and keeled scars are disappearing, some of which have been on my body for forty years. It is truly amazing." *H.M., California*

24. "After a motorcycle race, I suffered a serious third degree burn on my leg from an exposed exhaust pipe. The burn healed in less than one month, and in six weeks was just a dark spot. In the past, burns like this have taken six months to heal."

Others have reported a much clearer mind and more vivid memory. People have experienced more clear and active meditations. We have found that the Harmonizer causes an accelerated healing of cuts and wounds on the skin. It apparently is activating some cellular response as skin cuts seem to heal in a one quarter or less time than normal. The only negative aspect that we have found is that it pulls up emotional programs that have repressed in the past, and the person has to deal with them.

We hesitate to list many of the other results people have received so as not to create expectations, and we stress that the Harmonizer is only an *adjunct* to your body. You must work with it, and not expect it to do things for you. Please do not put unrealistic expectations on it as it's only a catalyst for your own healing miracles. You still have do your part in releasing the emotional trauma responsible for the health condition.

New Products and Upgrades

The price of the new 800 millivolt 9.216 MHz Body/Mind Harmonizer unit is $295.00 plus shipping. (If you have an old original 12.5 Hz or lower unit, we will exchange it for the 9.126 MHz unit and give you a trade-in value of $50.00.)

A new therapeutic unit is being developed that will have an adjustable power output, from 800-millivolts to 5-volts, *five times* more powerful than the current unit. Projected price is $395.00 or less depending on final cost.

A new "ghost buster" unit will be available soon for clearing buildings and creating an overall balancing/clearing effect in seminar and workshop facilities. Projected price is $450.00 or less depending on final cost.

We are working on a new unit that will operate on 120 volt AC house electricity. It will combine both units plus a programming mode to hook up with a tape recorder or a CD player for use with music and voice tapes for reprogramming the mind. One unit will have a tape recorder built into it. It will use piezo-electric discs similar to earphones to input information through the eighth cranial nerve. In this manner, it bypasses the Middle Self, which cannot then tamper or sabotage the input (all dysfunction of the body is mind controlled). In our tests, deaf people reported being able to hear the input, also. People have reported that they were able to learn a foreign language in as little as two weeks. A teacher reported that learning-disabled students were able to master lessons that they had not been able to in the past. Projected price on this unit is about $795.00 depending on final costs, and will include some programming software.

To order the Body/Mind Harmonizer, or books and tapes, call or write:

The Wellness Institute
8300 Rock Springs Rd.
Penryn, CA 95663
(800) 655-3846 (Orders only—all major credit cards accepted)
Fax: (916) 663-0134
E-mail: artmartin@mindspring.com
Websites: www.medicalelectronics.org
www.mindbodymedicineconnection.com
www.personaltransformationpress.com

Appendix C: Tapes and Books

The first two books are available in most bookstores in the U.S. and in some countries around the world. The other five are available in spiral bound pre-publication format from publisher, Personal Transformation Press.

2011: The New Millennium Begins
$13.95, ISBN 1-891962-02-7
What can we expect the future to bring? How do we handle the coming changes and what do we look for? Prophesy for future earth changes and new planet Earth as it makes the quantum jump from the third to the fifth dimension.

Becoming a Spiritual Being in a Physical Body
$14.95, ISBN 1-891962-03-5
The "operations manual" for your life. Recreating your life for peace, happiness, harmony, and joy. Changing from being a physical being having transitory spiritual experiences to becoming a spiritual being in a physical body. Letting go of the duality of life.

Journey Into The Light
$9.95, ISBN 1-891962-05-01
The process of ascension and the steps that govern the journey to a light being. Looking for the missing link in evolution. Stepping out of the cycle of reincarnation.

Recovering Your Lost Self
$14.95, ISBN 1-891962-08-6
The author's journey from victim to cause in his life. How you can find your true self and have abundance in your life. Accepting unconditional love in your life through forgiveness and acceptance. Coming to the point where peace, happiness, harmony and joy are reality, not an illusion.

Pychoneuroimmunology: The Body/Mind Medicine Connection
ISBN 1-891962-07-8
What is psychoneuroimmunolgy and the mind/body medicine connection? An overview of the modalities and processes. Integrating the concepts. Research on the modalities. The mind as network computer. Affirmations, software for the mind. Neuro-Kinesiology. Using muscle testing for clearing beliefs and concepts, pro-

grams, patterns and records that are causing allergies, emotional behavior patterns, disease, illness and physical breakdown in the body. Neuro/Cellular Repatterning, a method to access the mind's programs, beliefs and interpretations and release them to heal any disease, illness or dysfunction in the mind/body. Miracle healings on demand with love and forgiveness. Supporting the body with nutritional and herbal products.

Tapes

Tapes are available on the guided imagery to train yourself to access the records and on the process for contacting your teacher and accessing the Hall of Records.

1. The Seven Chakra Guided Imagery:
   Train yourself to step out of the body to enter the Temple and the Hall of Records.

2. Accessing your Akashic Records:
   On the process and the various forms and methods of finding the answers to all your questions.

3. Psycho/Physical Self Regulation:
   Originally a tape for runner and walkers to regulate, flush the body of toxins and burn fat for energy. Can be used to train yourself to eat properly and reduce weight.

About The Author

In today's world, the issue of credibility often comes up. How many degrees do you have? What colleges did you attend? Who did you study with? Who were your teachers? How do you know this works?

When I needed outside validation and acceptance, those were valid questions. Now I do not consider them valid, nor do I care if others reject me because I don't have the credibility they seek. What I learned in college has no relevance to what I do now in my practice. What I know is far more important than my background. Therefore, I am not interested in listing all my credentials.

Neuro/Cellular Repatterning is a process that was developed by myself and three people who worked with me during the research period: Dr. James Dorabiala, Mike Hammer and Bernard Eckes. And new information still pours in even today. This is basically a self-taught process, and everyone who worked with us over the last 20 years are our students and our teachers.

What *is* relevant is that we be open to new ideas. I will attend others' workshops and experience their treatments. Healing is an open-ended and ongoing process in which we need to be open to new ideas. The "sacred cow" syndrome is out-dated and does not work for me.

Someone once attacked me with, "You think you have the whole pie, don't you? You believe that nobody can match up to you."

My response was, " I don't think I have the whole pie, but based on the success of the last 20 years, maybe I have a few more pieces than some other practitioners."

Art was born into a family where his father wanted a child and his mother did not. As an only child, he did not have any sibling interaction, so his only contacts were at school. His dysfunctional family laid down many problems, which he has come a long way in clearing, thanks to discovery of the process he developed—Neuro/Cellular Repatterning—and the people who worked with him over the years.

In 1963, he quit college after five years feeling frustrated with the educational system. He dabbled in real estate, but found that it was not his calling. In 1965, he married Susie, his partner ever since. Their sons, Ross and Ryan, were born in 1971 and 1976.

Very few people in the field of therapy work seem to be able to stay in relationship due to the fact they do not want to deal with their own issues. Art was committed to find himself and went on a path to do so. He stabilized his own relationship by working out his issues.

In 1968, he and Susie found themselves in St. Helena, CA, rebuilding an abandoned winery. To clear the land to plant grapes, Art became a logger. To support his family while the winery was being rehabilitated, he hired out his D8 Caterpillar tractor for land-clearing and vineyard preparation. After seven years, the big money interests were pushing grape prices below what was economically viable for a small winery to stay in business, so he sold the winery.

His next venture was a restaurant which he built himself, but found that the restaurant field is one of the most demanding there are. Despite instant financial success, he sold the restaurant after four months and moved on. However, Art met his first teacher at the restaurant, someone who planted a seed of doubt about his life path. At the time, Art was trying to find himself and was studying extensively and attending self-improvement seminars. After closing time, they would spend many hours talking about their paths.

In 1978, the buyers of the restaurant went bankrupt, so their payments stopped. Art had to return to work and his quest was disrupted. Fortunately, Susie was working full-time, but in 1980, she was laid off and Art, who had a green thumb, worked as a gardener at a senior citizens' complex. Having closely studied the Findhorn community, he took the opportunity to apply what he had learned about the earth spirits. He found, from the plants themselves, that the landscape architect had put many of them in the wrong place. Over the next year, he transformed the barren grounds into magnificent flower gardens, and even built a passive solar greenhouse to grow flowers year around.

By 1982, his healing practice was established so he quit the gardener job and concentrated on researching healing practices.

Art soon found that Santa Rosa, CA did not support the type of work he was doing, and when Joshua Stone invited him to go to Los Angeles to give readings to clients, he jumped at the opportunity. He and Joshua found they worked well together as a team, and Art was able to provide a unique and valuable service to many therapists. However, the traveling almost broke up his family, so they moved to Sacramento, CA, and opened a bookstore and metaphysical center.

While Art received considerable support for this venture, he didn't anticipate that few people had the money to support it financially. Having invested all the family's savings, and refinanced their house, all went well for almost three years until he took on partners in order to expand. However, his partners did not understand the law of cause and effect, and when they embezzled $28,000, the business went under.

Knowing that "What goes around comes around," Art managed to accept what had happened, forgive them and get on with his life. However, trying to understand the lesson in this was hard to accomplish. When you are angry at losing your life savings and 20 years of hard work, the clarity and acceptance that he had set it all up came slowly. Even though he knew this at one level, it was a hard lesson to learn. The lesson was that while he received much verbal validation from those who supported the center, he was paying over half its operational costs.

The failure was a mixed blessing. It put him on a new path, one in which he traveled and spread the word of his work, and really had to get down to business. He did finally recover, even though they lost their house and one of their cars.

Looking back, Art recognizes the many great strides forward that he has made. Today, he travels extensively giving lectures, seminars and workshops on a variety of subjects. He also has a circuit of cities that he visits regularly for individual sessions.

He has set up a publishing company to promote his books (see list in the front of this book), and they are available through the Wellness Institute. Many of them will be in bookstores in 1999.

He can be reached at 1 800 OK LET GO (655-3846)